YOU’
ON
YOUR
OWN

A MEMOIR

LYNNETTE FRITSHAW

This book depicts actual events in the life of the author as truthfully as recollection permits and/or can be verified by research. The conversations in the book all come from the author's recollections, though they are not written to represent word-for-word transcripts, and may not reflect the perspectives of others. Rather, the author has retold them in a way that evokes the feeling and meaning of what was said and, in all instances, the essence of the dialogue is accurate. All persons within are actual individuals; there are no composite characters. No names of individuals have been used to respect their privacy.

ISBN paperback: 978-1-0690815-0-6
ISBN eBook: 978-1-0690815-1-3
ISBN hardcover: 978-1-0690815-2-0

Cover design by Lynnette Fritshaw
Photography by Kimberly Goodwin

Printed in Canada

For my son, Tasen—
You are my greatest joy, and my constant inspiration.
May you always have the courage to face your fears and chase your dreams.
I love you.

CONTENTS

INTRODUCTION

I dedicated eighteen years of my life to the fire service. Not only was this a profession; I had a heartfelt duty to serve and protect my community. From my humble beginnings as a paid-on call auxiliary member to my eventual transition into a full-time career firefighter, every moment I spent in service was imbued with a deep sense of pride and responsibility. Contrary to the common narrative, my journey into firefighting was far from conventional. Unlike many of my peers who harbored childhood dreams of donning the uniform, the idea of becoming a firefighter hadn't even crossed my mind during my formative years. There were no familial ties that bound me to the profession, nor was there a childhood aspiration fueled by movies and television shows. In fact, the notion of firefighting didn't even register on my radar until much later in life. To be honest, the calling was very random. Yet despite my unconventional path, once I found myself immersed in the world of firefighting, I discovered an extreme sense of pride and ownership that I hadn't encountered elsewhere. It was as though fate had led me to this vocation and unveiled a calling that resonated deeply within my soul.

"I can't even imagine the trauma you've endured from the things you've seen and done in your job" was a common comment I received from people.

It's true that I attended some extremely horrific scenes and dealt with highly stressful calls. Surprisingly, though, the trauma I experienced did not stem from those incidents . . . *yet.* While the potential for delayed emotional impact exists—trauma has a sneaky way of manifesting later in life—so far, that has not been my result.

My psychological injuries stemmed from toxic messaging I received as a child, navigating a multitude of toxic, abusive, and manipulative relationships, and concluded by enduring years of bullying, discrimination, misogyny, and harassment from men in authority positions in my career.

The fire service remains a male-dominated industry, with approximately 6 percent of career firefighters in Canada being female. I was the first and only female in my local fire department. Breaking into that entrenched culture and the "old boys club" was an incredibly challenging task. I wasn't prepared for just how difficult it would be or the significant toll it would take on me mentally, emotionally, and physically.

Trauma wasn't just what happened *to* me; it was what happened *inside* of me. Little by little, my experiences transformed everything about who I was and what I stood for. They changed the way I thought, the way I performed my job, and how I showed up in my daily life. Over time, I became unrecognizable to myself and suffered in silence for many years. I kept secrets to keep others comfortable, sacrificing my own well-being in the process. My job became my identity and I spent over a decade trying to prove myself worthy. I had convinced myself that the sacrifice and suffering would be worth it one day.

"One day" finally came but not in the form I expected. I chose to get really fucking honest with myself and acknowledge the role I was playing in my own suffering. Staying silent wasn't serving me; it was destroying me. I needed to find my voice, but first, I needed to heal. So I embarked on a healing journey that took me to the depths of my being and back again. I surrendered to the process and trusted myself for the first time in over a decade. It was hard and messy as fuck, but it wasn't nearly as painful as the suffering I had endured. I knew it would be worth it.

I reached a point where I couldn't progress any further in my healing journey without telling my story. Yet I couldn't tell my story while still being employed. So, I made the very difficult decision to take early retirement and step away from a career I deeply loved. I knew it was necessary to prioritize my well-being. For the first time in many years, I chose to put myself first, and it felt incredibly empowering.

Everything I experienced shaped who I am today. I am proud of the strength, courage, and resilience I brought forth, which kept me pushing forward, even during the darkest times. I used every stone thrown at me to build the steps from who I was to who I am now. I turned my wounds into wisdom and am now using my voice to impact the lives of others.

I don't have a secret; I have a story.

CHAPTER 1

Broken Foundation

"Do you want something to cry about?"

These words echoed throughout my childhood and often marked the beginning of harsh lessons that I wasn't ready to learn. Growing up, the line between discipline and emotional pain was blurred. Reprimands felt like an attack on my worth and left scars that would take years to understand—and even longer to heal.

I read a publication that stated a large majority of first responders have experienced childhood trauma. That revelation shed light on so much for me. Compounding trauma throughout my life, starting at an early age, predisposed me to failure. The only difference for me was that failure was never an option.

Experiencing childhood trauma laid the foundation and shaped the intricate formation of certain behavioral patterns throughout my life. These deeply engrained patterns, often subconscious, dictated my responses and decisions, influencing every aspect of my being. It wasn't until I chose to embark on a deep journey of self-discovery in my mid-forties that I began to unravel the complex web of experiences and suppressed emotions that had woven themselves into the fabric of my identity. This journey unveiled that I wasn't who I believed I was meant to be, and it became clear that reaching my true potential would require me to confront and battle the painful truths and demons of my past I had long avoided. Refusing to allow my past to dictate my future, I actively began reclaiming control of my narrative.

I was born and raised in Dawson Creek—a small town in northern British Columbia, Canada—where the economy is powered by agriculture, oil and gas, and its widely known as "mile zero" of the Alaska Highway. Over the years I have been asked to characterize my childhood and I have grappled with the complexities of my experiences. Some moments evoked memories of warmth and love within the confines of a nurturing home; others were tainted by the shadow of adversity and trauma in an environment rife with toxicity. I have found it very challenging to neatly categorize my upbringing while navigating between those contrasting realities. I'm a Generation Xer and this group embodies a unique blend of contrasting experiences in both technology and personal communication. Most would say I had a "normal" childhood, but what is normal with ever-changing definitions of the word?

There was a stark contrast between my parents' personalities, which ultimately led to their divorce before I reached my teenage years. Their separation brought its own set of challenges, making it both a blessing and a curse. The blessing was in the dissolution of their unhappy marriage, which was characterized by constant conflict and discord. However, the curse resulted from the lingering effects of their toxicity that persisted even in their absence from one another. All the memories of yelling, fighting, arguing, and the unsettling sounds of doors slamming and objects breaking punctuated my childhood and left indelible marks on my psyche. Some periods have been so deeply buried in my subconscious that I have blocked them out entirely. This coping mechanism shielded me from the trauma and allowed me to feel safe in the moment.

Lurking in the shadows, I secretly bore witness to a multitude of distressing situations that unfolded within the confines of my family. From the sidelines I watched my mother weather a relentless storm of mistreatment, unacceptable behaviors, and a variety of abuse throughout the years from my father. Unfortunately, I wasn't merely a passive observer. I, too, became a target of similar treatment on numerous occasions. These turbulent years were marked by an overwhelming sense of fear, insecurity, and perpetual uncertainty that cast a dark shadow over our household. Eventually the strain became unbearable and led to my parents' decision to separate. As they embarked on this tumultuous journey of separation, my brother and I remained anchored in our family home with our mother, while our father ventured out and began a new chapter elsewhere. The transition was dramatic and stressful. The pervasive cloud of confusion added even more uncertainty.

My mother embodied a relentless work ethic and was always juggling multiple jobs from sunup to sundown to ensure our family had the financial stability we needed. From the time I reached babysitting age, I took on the role of overseeing my younger brother and shouldering responsibilities beyond my years. Despite the weight of these obligations, I maintained a sense of responsibility and dependability because I knew that my mother needed my help so she could follow through with her obligations. I often resented the absence of my mother due to her demanding work schedule. Yet at the same time, I couldn't help but admire her unwavering determination and resilience. Despite facing seemingly insurmountable challenges, she always problem-solved, persevered, and found solutions to make ends meet and provide for our family. Her unyielding drive to overcome adversity left an indelible impression on me that instilled a profound respect for her strength and resourcefulness. Even in the face of adversity, she remained steadfast and continually demonstrated an unwavering commitment to ensuring our well-being and security.

My father's occupation as a truck driver meant he was often absent during my formative years. When he wasn't on the road, he frequently immersed himself in pleasure, such as playing in a band and indulging in alcohol-fueled social gatherings. His presence brought a mixture of excitement and vitality, but it also cast a shadow of apprehension and unease. Despite his jovial demeanor in social settings, I harbored a deep-seated fear of my father that was rooted in his volatile temper and tendency for excessive punishment. He had unpredictable outbursts that created a sense of wariness and caution in me and tarnished the "fun parent" image he sometimes portrayed. Beneath the surface, I longed for a nurturing and supportive relationship with him, but his selfishness and stubbornness created an emotional distance that seemed impossible to bridge. I was driven by an insatiable desire for validation and acceptance from my father, so I spent many years seeking his approval and hoping to earn his affection and recognition. Yet despite my efforts, most often our relationship was ridden with tension and unspoken resentment that left me grappling with feelings of inadequacy and longing for a connection that always seemed out of reach.

Establishing a meaningful connection with my younger brother has proven to be a constant struggle. His battle with addiction has cast a shadow over our relationship, and my heart aches for him to triumph over his demons. I have often found myself reflecting on our shared childhood and recognizing the ways in which our upbringing contributed to his current struggles. I wish I could rewind the clock to spare him from the pain and hardships that he has endured. Growing up I always felt that my brother was favored by our father, which fueled a lot of resentment within me. It appeared that he basked in our father's approval while I languished in the shadows. However, as the years passed, the dynamics of that relationship shifted dramatically. Our father's disappointment and disapproval became directed solely at my brother and led to his eventual disownment due to his destructive behaviors. The irony of that reversal was not lost on me. Despite the tumultuous nature of our relationship, I have never stopped hoping for my brother's redemption and recovery. His struggles have taught our family a lot about compassion and acceptance, and I wish for him to remain steadfast on his journey toward healing and wholeness.

Stretches of my childhood have remained elusive, even with my relentless efforts to summon them from the depths of my memory. I have been curious to piece together the fragments of my past and fill in the voids that have been left by the missing pieces. Yet despite my best attempts, the memories have remained stubbornly hidden. In stark contrast to the evasive memories, there have been a handful of vivid recollections that refuse to fade with time. They have served as haunting reminders of the pain and turmoil that once gripped my young heart and have left scars that have yet to fully heal.

I recall a seemingly ordinary day when I was six or seven, standing with my mother in the driveway as my father backed his truck onto the street. My little brother was seated beside him. What followed was anything but ordinary. As my father maneuvered the truck to the middle of the street, he suddenly shoved my brother's head out of the open driver's side window.

"Take a good look at him!" he uttered; the chilling words directed at my mother. "Because this is the last time you're ever going to see him!"

With that ominous declaration, my father sped off, leaving my mother and me stunned and bewildered. The scream that erupted from her pierced the air and was one I would never forget. It was a raw expression of panic and fear. In that moment, the world seemed to tilt on its axis, and I was gripped by a sense of profound uncertainty and dread. What transpired before or after that traumatic scene remains shrouded in mystery to me. I have no recollection of what led up to that moment or how the events unfolded afterward. It's as if the memory exists in isolation, disconnected from any context or resolution. My father obviously returned with my brother at some point, but I have struggled to make sense of the missing puzzle pieces. Even though I may never fully understand what happened that day, its impact on me was indelible.

A few years later my family and I were homebound in the car, but I can't recall where we were returning from. As we drove, tension filled the air as my parents engaged in a heated argument. As we watched the turmoil unfold, my brother and I sought solace by holding each other's hands tightly in the back seat. Suddenly, my father's anger escalated, and he abruptly pulled the car to a stop by the roadside. His shouts filled the interior as he reached across my mother, opened the passenger door, and forcibly attempted to eject her from the car. The forceful shoves slid my mother to the edge of her seat, where she teetered before tumbling out onto the ground. Panic gripped me as I struggled to quickly undo my seat belt and desperately reached out for my mother, fearing for her safety. Before my mother could fully remove her legs from inside the car, my dad recklessly let off the brake, heedless of her precarious position. I screamed in terror and hastily flipped her seat forward to free myself. My father was yelling at me to stay put, but I ignored his commands and leapt out of the car to join my mother on the roadside. He hollered at me to close the car door, so I gave it a weak push. As it shut, he sped away with my brother still in the back seat. My father had chosen to leave us stranded. Immediately, I felt a surge of abandonment and confusion.

I quickly gathered my wits and helped my mother to her feet. We were both in tears, but together we started on the daunting journey home by foot. Each step was heavy with the weight of uncertainty and fear. When we finally arrived at the house we were met with chaos. The once-familiar sanctuary of our home was now marred by destruction. Some walls bore the scars of punched holes, and the kitchen was in complete disarray, with the fridge sprawled face down on the floor. My mother and I immediately scoured the house to find my brother safe and unharmed. Not a word was exchanged between my mother and me; it wasn't necessary. With silent determination, we commenced the arduous task of restoring order to our shattered home. Though I knew my father was present somewhere in the house, the rest of what happened has remained obscured. Like the other memory, I may never fully piece the rest of the story together or understand that turbulent day, but I have been left with its impact imprinted forever.

Growing up witnessing and being exposed to the tumultuous dynamics of a relationship characterized by alcoholism, multiple forms of abuse, and infidelity provided a less-than-ideal foundation for my future success. The messages I received during my formative years were so damaging, as they shaped my perception of relationships and influenced my emotional development in profound ways. The absence of stability and the prevalence of destructive behaviors left a lasting impact. Unbeknownst to me at the time, that messaging created the belief systems I lived by until I made the conscious decision to start digging deep into myself and my shadows.

I had been programmed to give people a million chances and believed in them more than they believed in themselves. I tried to see the good in others and pushed through the bad, even when there was more bad than good. I allowed mistreatments and bad behavior to be excused by insincere apologies just to keep the peace. I set my worth and my value by the judgements of others and molded myself to meet their expectations and desires. I found fault in myself and took responsibility for the actions of others. I learned how to be extremely stubborn and get my own way. I would not take no for an answer and used force to get things to happen. I did not take ownership of my wrongdoings and failed to consider the needs and feelings of others. I learned how having a temper made me appear bigger and stronger. I learned that to be loved by others, I had to excuse their behaviors and accept mistreatment. I learned to portray a polished exterior and keep secrets behind closed doors.

On the positive side, I learned how to work hard and go after what I wanted. I mastered resilience, fortitude, and the ability to persevere through even the most challenging circumstances. I learned to have love and compassion for others even when they didn't deserve it, and how important "chosen" family was. I also learned that consistent practice would get me results. That drive and determination would take me places. I learned that I could make mistakes and try again because the only way I would fail was if I quit.

The messaging I received was potent yet contradicting at times. I thought I had a clear understanding of what I wished to avoid in my life, but the influences of my childhood conditioning subtly guided me toward patterns and environments that mirrored those very things I sought to evade.

As I matured, I found myself pushing boundaries and embracing a rebellious streak in my teenage years. Despite the limits I tested, I somehow managed to navigate it all reasonably unscathed and escape the consequences of my actions. That period of my life unfolded in an era before cell phones and the internet, and for that I am sincerely thankful. In the absence of constant digital surveillance, I had the freedom to explore, make mistakes, and learn very valuable lessons without the scrutiny—or digital memory—of social media.

Although I possessed the smarts, my academic performance in school didn't reflect my potential and that was largely due to a lack of dedication and prioritizing my social life over schoolwork. Despite that, I managed to meet the necessary requirements and graduated high school alongside my friends. I had taken future planning programs but was uncertain about my desired career path. Instead of attending post-secondary school, I opted to enter the workforce immediately after graduation. I was confident that my experiences would eventually lead me to what I wanted to be when I grew up. Following graduation, I was eager to embrace independence and embark on the next chapter of my life, so I took the leap with my best friend, and we moved into our first apartment together. I was on my own and had to sustain myself financially, so that meant juggling two jobs simultaneously. I was driven by a strong work ethic and possessed a genuine appreciation for the value of hard-earned money. It required some hustle and some struggle to balance multiple responsibilities, but that didn't deter me. I was fueled by a determination to succeed.

After a few years of exploration, I reached a pivotal moment of clarity where I identified that my passion was hairstyling. I was always the go-to stylist for my friends, and I loved having the chance to experiment with creativity and artistic impression. The hands-on nature of the work gave me immense satisfaction especially when I could transform someone's appearance and boost their confidence.

I made the bold choice to further my education by enrolling in cosmetology school that was commencing the following week in another city a short distance away. I completely uprooted my life in a matter of a few days to follow my calling. Ten months later I successfully completed my training and eagerly immersed myself in the vibrant atmosphere of a renowned salon where I was able to hone my skills and gain invaluable experience. However, I soon felt compelled to forge my own path in the industry and took the leap into entrepreneurship. I possessed unwavering confidence and a vision for success, so it didn't take long before I took a huge risk and founded my own salon. I set off on a journey to carve my niche in the competitive beauty industry and began a thrilling chapter of solidifying my place in the hairstyling world.

Throughout my twenties, I was on a journey of self-discovery and eagerly explored new avenues and embraced every opportunity with go-getter energy. I had a fearless attitude toward challenges and thrived by taking risks. In my youthful confidence I viewed rejection as merely a temporary setback, which allowed me to approach everything with a steadfast belief in my abilities. Venturing into entrepreneurship proved to be the perfect outlet for my passion and determination, and it catapulted me into a realm where I flourished as a highly successful hairstylist and salon owner for an impressive fifteen-year tenure. That chapter of my life stood as a testament to the remarkable rewards that I could achieve by daring to dream big and persistently pursue my ambitions.

Throughout those periods I was involved in a couple of unsuccessful long-term committed relationships, as well as a couple of fast-and-dirty relations. I was easily sucked into intense whirlwind romances that escalated quickly. There was lack of communication in every relationship, frequent arguments, and a roller coaster of highs and lows. I continually subjected myself to connections that involved a series of lies, deceit, manipulation, and emotional turmoil. Every time I walked away; I left a trail of unresolved emotions dragging behind me.

As I reached the milestone of turning thirty, I felt a profound shift within myself. Despite being ahead of the curve, I found myself grappling with what felt like a premature midlife crisis. I had a deep yearning for greater fulfillment and purpose in my life. I needed and wanted more for myself. This need for more stemmed from a deeper desire to seek out meaning that would resonate on a soul level. It felt almost selfish to admit but the longing for a more purposeful existence gnawed at me and could not be ignored.

I was in a long-term committed relationship and on the brink of marriage, but even though we portrayed the appearance of stability and contentment, there lingered an undeniable void, and a vital element was missing. I couldn't shake the feeling of emptiness that pervaded that aspect of my life, but I had continued to push through it. It was as though a crucial piece of the puzzle was absent, and the relationship failed to provide me with the fulfillment and completeness that I yearned for. Here I was, faced with the tumult of a midlife crisis, so I made the conscious decision to focus my energies on addressing one facet at a time. While the relationship provided a semblance of comfort and stability, it was my career that I sensed held the key to unlocking a more gratifying existence. The path ahead was unknown and I struggled with ambiguity regarding the direction I should take. Nonetheless, I had a fierce determination burning within me to pursue a newfound sense of purpose and fulfillment in my professional pursuits.

My innate drive for physical activity and my deep-seated passion for helping others had long been defining aspects of my identity. While my career in the beauty industry allowed me to fulfill the latter, I wanted a way to leverage my physical prowess more effectively. Standing tirelessly behind a salon chair with my arms raised for hours on end and being bent over a sink multiple times a day took a huge toll on my body. It painfully manifested as chronic discomfort in my lower back and shoulders. It became apparent that I wanted to align my professional path more closely with my physical capabilities.

After some deliberation it seemed only natural to gravitate toward pursuing certifications in personal training and nutrition, as it was a realm that was already intertwined with my daily life and passions. I was not only making a strategic move toward safeguarding my physical well-being, but I was also directing a seamless integration of my innate strengths in a career path that promised to be both rewarding and fulfilling.

I made a decision and acted immediately, making obtaining both certifications happen swiftly. I harmoniously integrated personal training sessions into my schedule on my days off and carved out time between my hairstyling clients. It was proving to be immensely gratifying. I was forging connections with clients and witnessing their progress toward achieving their fitness aspirations. There was a sincere sense of fulfillment and gratification ignited within me. Working closely with individuals and guiding them along their wellness journeys didn't feel like a job; it was a passion.

I thrived in that environment for a couple of years, wholeheartedly dedicated to promoting health and well-being. I was surrounded by like-minded individuals who shared my zeal for fitness, and I relished the camaraderie and sense of purpose that permeated my days. Yet despite the undeniable fulfillment derived from my role, an underlying restlessness persisted; a nagging feeling that something vital remained unfulfilled. As rewarding as it was, that chapter of my life failed to encompass the entirety of what I sought and left me with a yearning for a deeper, more profound sense of purpose and alignment.

CHAPTER 2

Good Thing I'm Not A Lady

I remained on the hunt for that elusive "it." After an extensive period of exploration, I unexpectedly stumbled upon the realm of fire investigation and its intricacies immediately piqued my interest. The investigative aspect tapped into my natural curiosity and penchant for uncovering the truth—I could be quite the private investigator when I sensed something was amiss.

I knew absolutely nothing about firefighting, so I researched the interplay between fire investigation and the firefighting profession. I went on a mission to unravel the symbiotic relationship between the two fields. As I delved deeper into my inquiries, I realized there may be potential value in possessing firsthand knowledge of firefighting operations to enhance my efficacy as a fire investigator. I toyed with the notion that critical evidence could possibly be obscured during firefighting procedures and that spurred me to consider the benefits of understanding both disciplines. What began as a mere brainstorming session quickly evolved into a proactive pursuit of knowledge and skill enhancement. Being an action taker, I swiftly acted on what I deemed the logical next step. I started researching fire investigation courses, found one that I felt was best suited for me, and by weeks end had enrolled myself. It was literally *that* fast! With the groundwork laid, I launched into the next phase of my exploration and sought to glean insights from my local fire department in hopes of obtaining firsthand knowledge from those who were entrenched in the profession.

The firehall was a mysterious place to me, as it was a realm I had never ventured into before. Unlike many children who fondly recalled school tours or impromptu visits to admire the gleaming fire trucks, I had never set foot inside one. In fact, it wasn't until I mustered the courage to pick up the phone and inquire about visiting that I realized just how little I knew about this public service building. The voice on the other end of the phone informed me that the firehall was indeed open to the public at any time and I didn't need an appointment. That revelation alone underscored my lack of knowledge about this unfamiliar domain.

A couple of days later, I mustered the courage to step foot inside the firehall and braced myself for the unknown. As I crossed the threshold, my eyes swept over the surroundings and took in all the sights and sounds of the unfamiliar territory. I was promptly greeted by two men who were clad in the unmistakable uniform of firefighters. With a tentative smile, I shook their hands, introduced myself, and explained to them the purpose of my visit. Much to my dismay, the initial warmth I had received was quickly replaced by a visible shift in both of their demeanors. Immediately, their expressions hardened, and a wave of skepticism washed over them as I explained my intentions. In an instant, they made their disapproval of my pursuits clear and delivered blunt and opinionated statements that seemed intent on discouraging me from pursuing any angle of firefighting as a career.

"Firefighting is not a job for a lady," one guy informed me. "Nor is the firehall a place for one either."

Being the smart-ass that I was, I met his resistance head-on and refused to be swayed by his antiquated notions of gender roles. I retorted with a quick-witted comeback.

“It’s a good thing I’m not a lady,” I replied with a hint of defiance.

Being complete strangers, I had hoped to lighten the concern by injecting a dose of playful banter into the tense exchange. It brought a slight smile to their faces but not much else. Even though there was obvious friction, I remained steadfast in my plan to gather information that would better inform my decision regarding my future career path. Much to their dismay, I chose to remain on the premises because I was determined to find answers to my many questions and gain deeper insight. Their annoyance was palpable as I refused to be deterred. One of them informed me curtly that answering my questions was not their responsibility and instructed me to wait while they found someone more suitable. They departed in opposite directions and left me standing alone in the entryway for a lengthy period. Eventually, one of the men returned and informed me that I should take my questions to the fire chief. He pointed toward an office and then walked away without another word. Left alone once again, I cautiously made my way in the direction he had indicated.

As I approached the office door, the fire chief stood from behind his desk and welcomed me warmly. He approached with his hand extended and greeted me with a firm handshake. After we introduced ourselves, he gestured for me to sit in one of the chairs opposite his desk. I began to explain the purpose of my visit, much as I had to the others, but this time I was met with a smile and genuine interest. The fire chief listened attentively as I laid out my questions. He answered each one thoroughly and provided some valuable insights and practical advice. His demeanor was encouraging and supportive and put me at ease. After addressing all my queries, he concluded with words of encouragement, which were a welcome surprise. I thanked him sincerely for his time and assistance before leaving the firehall. As I walked away, I felt a twinge of excitement knowing I had just taken a deliberate step toward carving out a path that would be uniquely my own.

When it came to firefighter training, I found myself confronted with a plethora of options, and each one promised to equip me with the skills and knowledge that were necessary to be successful in the field. After careful consideration of my circumstances, I opted to enroll in a fire academy that offered a flexible approach to learning. This particular program allowed me to complete the theoretical coursework from the comfort of my own home and utilize online resources and exams to assess my understanding of the material. Following that, I would be partaking in a two-week intensive practical segment and writing my final exams at an academy located in Texas. The major appeal of this arrangement was its compatibility with my existing commitments and responsibilities. As the owner of a thriving business and a homeowner, I was juggling a myriad of adult responsibilities on the daily. The flexibility afforded by the online component of the course enabled me to strike a realistic balance between work, leisure, and study. I could easily integrate my studying into the after-hours of my busy schedule, which would allow me to maximize efficiency without compromising on the quality of my education. This approach excited me because it not only accommodated the demands of my professional and personal life, but it also empowered me to pursue my aspirations without undue disruption.

While working through my studies, I found myself veering off course and being drawn into a compelling investigation of women's representation in the fire service. To my astonishment, I uncovered a stark reality: only a mere 6 percent of career firefighters in Canada were female. This eye-opening revelation not only served as a reminder of the vast gender disparity that pervaded the profession, but also the depth of my own ignorance regarding the field of firefighting. I would never have guessed that female presence in the profession was that low. With a newfound sense of curiosity sparked, I ventured on a quest into the historical and regional context of women's involvement in firefighting. To my surprise, I discovered another startling revelation: my local fire department had *never* employed a female firefighter in a career capacity. In fact, according to the information I unearthed, the entire northern region of British Columbia had yet to witness a woman donning the uniform in a full-time capacity. Now that piqued my interest and had my full attention! This surprising fact sparked a firestorm of questions for me and ignited a demand to uncover the underlying reasons behind this glaring absence of female representation. I made a mental note to broach this topic during my next visit to the firehall.

Some of my classmates were discussing their involvement as volunteers and paid-on-call auxiliary members in their local fire departments, and how they were aiming to gain practical experience to improve their chances of securing full-time positions. I had never heard of that and was intrigued, so I decided to explore that avenue for myself in hopes that it could complement my textbook knowledge.

I ventured back to my local department and, as luck would have it, was met by the same two men I had talked to previously. They seemed just as eager to view me through the same lens as last time. I told them I was there to inquire about their auxiliary program and was immediately met with strong opposition and discriminatory remarks. One of them "kindly" reminded me that the firehall was no place for a woman, then followed it up by telling me that my presence would only invite trouble.

Unbeknownst to them, their response unwittingly shed light on my impending question of why there had never been a female firefighter at that location before. I couldn't help but notice the disdain in their tone. It wasn't the playful banter I had initially excused it as; it was downright disrespectful and plain fucking rude. My intention was simple. I was looking to volunteer my time and learn about the profession. Nothing more, nothing less. Yet their uncultured remarks tainted the atmosphere. My interest in auxiliary firefighting was by no means being driven by passion; rather, it felt like a necessary step toward my goal of becoming a fire investigator. So despite their discouraging comments and hostile demeanor, I chose to ignore them for selfish reasons. I needed the experience, and this avenue seemed like the most practical means for me to attain it.

Becoming an auxiliary firefighter required completing an application package that would be followed by an interview process. After submitting my application, I found myself in a waiting game as the progress toward the interview phase was moving at a painfully slow pace. I was eager to gain some practical experience while awaiting the next step, so I approached the deputy fire chief and asked for permission to attend the weekly Tuesday night practices. My schooling timeline was ticking away, and I was keen to get some hands-on experience before I departed for Texas. Thankfully, permission was granted. So I began showing up faithfully every Tuesday night. On more than one occasion, the on-duty captain pulled me aside before practice and made it very clear that I was to remain passive. I was told to stay out of the way. I was only allowed to observe. And I was not to touch anything. My eagerness to learn and participate was dampened by being sidelined but I did what was demanded. Even though it felt degrading, I stood off to the side with my hands behind my back as I had been relegated to the role of silent observer. I was allowed to exist on the periphery where I was to be seen and not heard. Even the questions I dared to ask were met with a look of annoyance and then ignored.

Of course, the dynamic of the Tuesday practice nights often varied due to the rotating crews and offered me glimpses of hope amidst the consistent challenges. On fortunate occasions, I encountered captains who welcomed my presence beyond mere attendance and fostered an environment where not only were my questions acknowledged and answered but my participation was actually encouraged. There were some supportive leaders and fellow auxiliaries who created a valuable learning opportunity by taking the time to personally guide me through the intricacies of operating unfamiliar equipment. On several occasions I brought my school textbook to practice night and was armed with questions from my studies. When I knew the practice was being led by certain captains, I seized the chance to seek clarification and witness firsthand demonstrations on any concepts I found puzzling. Their guidance and willingness not only bridged the gap between theory and practice, but it also deepened my understanding of firefighting principles in a tangible, hands-on manner that I needed.

After patiently waiting, I finally received the long-awaited invitation for an interview, and it was scheduled to take place in the upstairs classroom at the firehall. As I entered the room, I found myself facing a panel comprised of the fire chiefs, a union representative, and a seasoned captain. The atmosphere was undeniably intimidating, but I refused to give it any attention and was determined to give them the best interview possible. I confidently answered a series of standard questions as I was reasonably prepared. Then came a question I was pretty sure no one else was asked.

"You would be the only woman here," the seasoned captain stated. "Do you feel comfortable with that?"

I responded without hesitation, knowing that this man had a daughter who was also working her way into a male-dominated industry. I stated that I believed he could personally relate to the familiar space I was in, to which he smiled and acknowledged that he could.

With that, my interview concluded. I stood, shook hands with everyone, offered my thanks, and expressed my eagerness to hear from them.

Shortly after the interview process commenced, I was invited to become an auxiliary firefighter.

I was eager and brimming with anticipation to embark on this new chapter toward enhancing my knowledge in firefighting to be of value in my quest of becoming a fire investigator. However, my excitement was quickly dampened as I faced the first hurdle of getting fitted with turnout gear. As I slipped into the protective gear that was intended to shield me from hazardous environments, it became painfully clear that it was not designed for the female body. The sizing and fit were nowhere near accurate proportions, and doubts crept in about the uniform's ability to adequately safeguard me during training and firefighting operations. I gently expressed my reservations and was met with dismissive remarks that this was all they had, and that if I wasn't satisfied, then perhaps this wasn't the right path for me.

Reluctantly, I soldiered on and made do with ill-fitting hand-me-down gear that failed to provide the level of protection I believed I needed. The issue persisted when it came to the self-contained breathing apparatus (SCBA) masks. Each one I tried on was disproportionately large for my face and resulted in significant air leakage and the risk of contaminated air infiltration. Their response? I was told to simply pull the straps tighter. But no matter how hard I tightened the straps on the headpiece, it didn't help. I made earnest attempts to address the safety concerns, but my voiced apprehensions were only misconstrued and taken as complaints. After much frustration, I sought the advice of one of the captains I felt comfortable with, and he confirmed that I could not safely wear the masks that were provided. He graciously assisted in finding me an SCBA mask that was marginally smaller, although still not an ideal fit. There were no further options presented, so I resigned myself to making the best of the situation and accepted that this was the beginning of my adaptation in having to "make do" with circumstances.

Now that I was an officially recognized auxiliary firefighter, I anticipated a shift in the dynamics of practice nights. I envisioned myself being fully integrated into the team, actively participating, and absorbing invaluable lessons along the way. While this scenario occasionally unfolded as I had hoped, the reality often fell short of my expectations. Regardless of my newfound status, there were still instances where certain captains told me that I was a liability and relegated me back to the role of a passive observer with strict instructions not to touch anything. In the odd occurrence when I was allowed to participate, there were frustrating limitations imposed upon me. If there were training drills involving SCBA, I found myself barred from using the carbon fiber air cylinders because they were lighter in weight. Instead, I was directed to only use the cumbersome steel ones. I was told that if I wanted to do the job, then I wasn't going to be getting any special treatment. I hadn't realized that a lighter air cylinder meant I was vying for some kind of special treatment. Certain individuals often went to great lengths to impose additional obstacles and hurdles and ensure that I didn't receive any advantages. I received plenty of special treatment from them, all right, but it was by no means in my favor.

On the contrary! There were a couple of captains who were the absolute opposite spectrum.

One evening during a training session, the piercing tones rang and the firefighter in charge of dispatching notified everyone that there were alarms ringing at a nearby school. The on-duty captain beckoned a couple of us auxiliaries to join them in the firetruck and respond to the call. Having the opportunity to be part of the action filled me with exhilaration. But as we sped away from the firehall, the flashing lights and blaring siren greatly intensified my anticipation. When we arrived on the scene, I shadowed the experienced crew closely and absorbed every detail of their actions. I watched as they meticulously assessed the situation while verbalizing their procedures and objectives. I was hungry for knowledge and hung on to their every word, soaking in the invaluable insights and the wealth of experience they were willing to share. As we wrapped up our duties at the scene, we made our way back to the truck for the return drive to the firehall.

"You're driving," the captain said to me nonchalantly, offering a slight smile.

I stopped dead in my tracks. Was he serious? He was willing to entrust me with the responsibility of driving? I was in sheer disbelief! Me? Behind the wheel of a fire truck? Holy fuck! Yes, please! It felt like a surreal privilege and my heart raced with excitement at the prospect. I climbed up into the driver's seat and looked around at the array of unfamiliar controls and gauges. My sense of awe and nervousness was heightened. With wide eyes, I glanced over at the captain, who was now occupying the passenger seat. His expression was a mix of encouragement and amusement as he gave me a nod and a side eye.

"Do you know what you're doing?" he asked, knowing full well by the look of terror and confusion on my face that I didn't.

"I absolutely do not," I replied with a nervous laugh.

He responded with a reassuring chuckle, then offered calm and detailed instructions as he guided me through each step of the process. The next thing I knew, we were moving, and I couldn't believe what was happening. I was actually driving a fire truck!

It was a winter scene, and the snowflakes were aggressively falling on the roads already cloaked in a layer of ice. I was navigating the truck through the treacherous conditions with intensity and caution. The captain fully recognized the conditions and provided verbal guidance on how to utilize the insta-chains for enhanced traction. He also emphasized the importance of understanding the size and dimensions of the truck so I would remember to take wider turns to safely maneuver around the slick streets and avoid the unforgiving curbs. I had both hands firmly gripping the wheel, and my eyes were laser-focused on the road ahead as I listened closely to every word of the captain's instructions on how to navigate the snow-covered streets with the utmost care. Even though there were unique challenges posed by the winter weather, I executed each turn mindfully and with precision. As we approached the firehall, I followed the captain's guidance meticulously and smoothly guided the truck onto the ramp and expertly backed it toward the entrance as instructed. We made it! As I brought the truck to a halt, the captain directed me to open the bay door and put the truck away. I was instantly overtaken with a wave of self-doubt!

"You want me to maneuver this massive truck through that tiny door backwards?" I blurted out, my uncertainty palpable.

He calmly replied, "Yes, that is what I want."

He then proceeded to offer a steady stream of instructions on how to align the tires with the reflective lines on the floor, to proceed slowly, and to remain vigilant by monitoring my mirrors. My nerves felt like a tangled knot, so I briefly hesitated to mentally map out the maneuver. I glanced repeatedly at the mirror and the reflective lines on the ground as I meticulously planned each step before mustering the courage to engage the truck in reverse. My internal turmoil was interrupted by the captain's reassuring voice as he nudged me to begin.

"You can do it," he stated, confident in my abilities.

Those simple yet profound words echoed in my mind and served as a beacon of encouragement as I realized, in that moment, the significance of his trust and belief in me.

Summoning my courage, I drew in a deep breath and shifted the truck into reverse. My eyes were fixated on the reflective lines on the floor through the mirror as I slowly released my foot from the brake and allowed the truck to start rolling backwards. Remarkably, on my very first attempt, I seamlessly backed the truck into its designated spot as if I had been doing it for years. With my foot firmly reapplied to the brake, I let out an exhale. I didn't even realize I had been holding my breath the entire time. My attention quickly switched to the captain's voice as I was now getting a new set of instructions. He had me transition the truck into neutral, engage the airbrakes, turn off the engine, and then power down the truck.

A surge of pride washed over me as I basked in the satisfaction of a job well done. It felt amazing. Everyone assisted as we diligently cleared the snow from the truck and the floor, ensuring everything was tidy and prepared for the next call. Once completed, we carried on with our training session. I glanced admiringly at the truck a few times and silently congratulated myself on not only being trusted to drive the truck, but for successfully completing the task. I realized the immense satisfaction that came from exceeding my own expectations.

As soon as I arrived home that night, I told my husband and my family what I had done. I was overflowing with excitement and couldn't contain the thrill of my accomplishment. I was eager to share the news with the girls and my clients at the salon the following day.

A new day dawned and the celebratory conversations at the salon were interrupted with a phone call. As I answered, I was met with a familiar voice that was devoid of any pleasantries and got straight to the point.

"Did you drive the truck last night?" the captain demanded to know.

My heart, which had soared with pride just hours before, now plummeted with apprehension. With a trembling voice I managed to stammer out a hesitant "yes," which was immediately met with a barrage of aggression on the other end of the line. His tone was harsh and packed with accusations, opinions, and thinly veiled threats. It went on for what felt like an eternity. Each word was a verbal assault that left very little room for breaths to be taken or any rebuttal. And then, just as abruptly as it had begun, the conversation ended with a sharp click on the other end of the line as he hung up on me. I stood there holding the phone and reeling in disbelief and confusion.

I could feel panic jolting through my body and tightening like a vice. Uncertainty flooded my mind as I tried desperately to pinpoint exactly what I had done wrong. There had been a multitude of harsh words and threats thrown my direction. It left me consumed by a shadow of doubt and fear. I had no idea what to do next. A storm of emotions swirled within me, and I felt like I was going to be sick. I quickly reached out to a captain whom I trusted implicitly and told him I was desperate for some guidance. I poured out the details of the distressing encounter and awaited his response with bated breath. He muttered a few words about the caller's lack of decency and respect and summed it up that the guy was simply an asshole, and I shouldn't worry about it.

I knew his words held truth, but they failed to ease my persistent worry. I thanked him for his time and hung up the phone. The worry remained in the forefront and weighed heavily on my thoughts for days. The time passed without any further mention of the matter from anyone, but I found very little solace in the absence of news. I deeply hoped that no news meant good news, yet I couldn't help but feel skeptical and insecure about that theory. Some days later, I finally received a call from the fire chief that brought some clarity amidst the uncertainty. He gave me a recount of the chaotic meetings that had happened since I'd parked the truck, where opinions clashed and some tempers flared, but assured me of my innocence. He advised with a note of caution against ever driving the truck again as an auxiliary, even if the captain deemed it permissible. He continued that with such discord among members and conflicting views prevailing, it was probably best to take the safest course and abstain from things like that entirely. I wholeheartedly agreed with him and felt a sense of relief wash over me. I was thankful to know that I wasn't in trouble or up against disciplinarily action of some sort. The call closed by him informing me that there were still a couple of men who weren't satisfied with the outcome as they had wanted me removed from the auxiliary program, but I could be reassured that wasn't happening.

Over the next couple of weeks, I was aggressively confronted on multiple occasions.

"You'd better learn your place—and quickly!" one man threatened. "And don't you dare try another stunt like that, or I promise there will be consequences next time."

Two of them cornered me and went so far as to suggest that resigning from my auxiliary position would be a face-saving measure for me before I was fired. I was devastated that it had turned into what it did. I never meant to upset anyone and I sure as hell hadn't done it without permission. But I went to great lengths to assure them that I would follow orders and never step out of line by driving the fire truck again. Even though I promised I had learned my lesson, they were relentless in reminding me of their authority position and how as an auxiliary, I was a nobody. The whole ordeal had me so consumed with worry and fear over looming potential consequences that I sought counsel from a few individuals I trusted. Their words echoed with solidarity as they assured me that resigning was unnecessary, and the possibility of expulsion was far-fetched considering the event.

Amidst all the turmoil, the captain who had granted me the privilege of driving the fire truck stepped forward and affirmed that the decision for me driving the truck rested solely on his shoulders. He was completely unshaken and unaffected by the chaos.

"I can do whatever the fuck I want," he boldly stated. "I couldn't care less what they say or think."

He advised me to do the same.

I wished I could have been as unbothered by the event as he advised but I continued to stress about it for an obscene amount of time. I kept looping back to one of the tongue-lashings where it was stated that I had shown them I couldn't be trusted and that I should be ashamed of myself. I prided myself on being a trustworthy person and felt ashamed of myself for letting them down. Overloaded with guilt and shame, I attempted to mend bridges. I offered numerous apologies to those who felt aggrieved, repeatedly pledging that I was trustworthy and would prove it to them to regain their trust. They refused to hear me, so I vowed to show them. Actions speak louder than words, so I peacefully accepted that there was no fucking way I would ever occupy the driver's seat again.

Despite the efforts of those select few to tarnish my experience, I silently clung to one high point. As wrong as my actions may or may not have been, the memory of driving the truck that night has always been something I've cherished and valued as an impressive accomplishment.

CHAPTER 3

Igniting Dreams

After diligently completing my home studies, I was officially prepared to embark on my journey to Texas for the two-week practical phase of my training and the completion of my final exams. In true fashion, I overpacked for the trip and set off with my conspicuously oversized bright-pink suitcase. Living in northern Canada meant I'd have to endure an excruciatingly long day of travel. After multiple flights, layovers, and customs, I finally arrived safe and sound. As anticipated, it had taken the entire day and was well into the night when I arrived, so I made my way to the hotel I had reserved. I was exhausted, laid my head down on the pillow, and stared at the ceiling, wide awake. I needed to sleep but the chances of that seemed impossible because I was brimming with anticipation and eagerness for the coming day. I had plenty of time the next morning to relax and prepare for my arrival at the academy, so I took advantage of it. After checking out of the hotel, I made my way to the academy and was one of the first to arrive. I welcomed the others as they filtered in throughout the day. I couldn't help but notice that amidst a sea of twenty-four men, I stood as the sole female in my cohort. Initially, that sparked a sense of unease and intimidation, but those feelings soon dissipated as I discovered the warmth and camaraderie shared among us as we were all united for the same purpose.

The academy was a fire station that boasted an impressive array of facilities. On the main floor were expansive truck bays that housed a gleaming fire engine, while adjacent spaces featured a well-appointed kitchen, complete with a spacious dining area, along with a large classroom and multiple administrative offices.

Ascending the stairs to the upper level revealed the sleeping quarters in a singular, cavernous room that was outfitted with rows of bunk beds. There were separate washrooms for men and women, which put me in the possession of a small victory. Even though it was exclusively mine to use, I willingly extended the invitation to my male counterparts to utilize it once I had completed my routine every morning and evening. Twenty-four of them waiting to use their bathroom when mine was empty felt unjust. Their gratitude was palpable as their respectful demeanor and diligent cleanliness didn't go unnoticed. Without having to say a word, they consistently cleaned up after themselves and left the space as immaculate as they found it.

The daily routine adhered to a very stringent schedule that instilled the core values of discipline and organization within the fire service. I eagerly rose from my bunk at the break of dawn each day to go outside and complete a workout. It consisted of running laps around the building, push-ups, jumping jacks, tire flips, and a variety of other miscellaneous exercises, followed by stretching. I reveled in the invigorating warmth of Texas in November. It was a stark contrast to the chill of home, as was the occasional surprise appearance of a scorpion.

Following the morning workout session, we would all gather to consume a hearty breakfast that was skillfully prepared to fuel our bodies for the challenging day ahead. As a group we were responsible for the subsequent cleanup and chores throughout our stay to reinforce the ethos of shared responsibility, which mirrored the duties that were to be expected in the real-life setting of a fire station.

Throughout the day, a blend of skills practice and classroom instruction kept me engaged and focused on honing my abilities and expanding my knowledge base. I was so thankful to have received hands-on experience at my local department prior to arriving. As evening descended each day, we would all gather in the dining hall for supper and then collectively complete another round of cleanup duties before dedicating ourselves to a few hours in the classroom for exam preparation.

Despite the exhaustive nature of the days—punctuated by long hours of study and intense physical exertion—I was filled with an undeniable sense of exhilaration. Extensive team-building exercises were incorporated into the training that fostered a spirit of camaraderie and mutual support. We worked hard together through the challenges and celebrated each triumph as a collective victory. It felt amazing to be part of such a tight-knit community, and the bonds I forged with my classmates were not only professional but deeply personal. There was a profound satisfaction in being respected, accepted, and belonging to a team.

Class concluded earlier than expected one day, and the instructors granted us the rare freedom to venture off-campus and indulge in our own pursuits. With a playful quip, one of the instructors suggested that I might fancy the mall for some shopping; others made plans to head for the gun range. There was no way this Canadian girl was taking in retail therapy and passing up the thrilling opportunity of firing handguns and machine guns! IYKYK. Even though my upbringing involved guns and hunting, I never had the opportunity to shoot handguns, so I was very excited to seize the moment. I eagerly accepted the invitation to join the group at the gun range. I think the guys were a little surprised at my selection and enthusiasm but happily welcomed me along. We spent the greater part of the afternoon experimenting with various firearms and comparing our marksmanship. The atmosphere crackled with friendly banter and competition, and I was delighted to prove my precision capabilities with each target comparison. The impromptu excursion away from the rigors of academy life was an unexpected yet invaluable team experience for me. I was grateful for the inclusion and will always cherish the memories that were forged amidst the echoing gunfire and camaraderie that day.

Every moment of my two-week stint at the fire academy in Texas was an absolute thrill. Being immersed in the experience ignited a passion within me that I didn't even know was there. I fell in love with the teamwork. I fell in love with the adrenaline rush. I fell in love with the ability to help others. And I downright fell in love with firefighting. Every aspect of it captivated my spirit, and I was fucking good at it too! I thrived at the physical challenges, earned leadership roles, pushed myself to set new benchmarks in timed events, and volunteered for the daring task of scaling the one-hundred-foot aerial ladder. The view from the top was breathtaking! I accepted every challenge without fear and was fueled by an unshakeable belief in my abilities. In those moments I was a force to be reckoned with and utterly unstoppable.

The fire academy training was drawing near, and my nerves were fluttering as my anticipation mounted for the final exams. I held a deep-seated confidence because I had studied my ass off and committed most of the material to memory. Moreover, the collective efforts we had demonstrated as a cohesive unit gave me a sense of assurance that we were all more than prepared to ace the exams. We wished each other luck for good measure even though I knew we didn't need it. I completed each part of the exam and then sat with the group as we awaited our individual results. The atmosphere was charged with a mix of jittery energy and subdued anticipation. Some paced anxiously while others sat in quiet contemplation, suppressing their inner turmoil. With each passing moment, I could feel the tension mounting until one by one we received the news that our hard work had paid off. I had passed all of my exams with flying colors! I was so insanely proud of myself and took a second to absorb the news.

The culmination of our journey was marked by a poignant graduation ceremony, which was a fitting tribute to our collective achievements. Tears welled in my eyes as I stood among my classmates, overflowing with pride not only for my own accomplishments but for the shared victories of those beside me. I was surrounded by dear friends who had become like family, and I realized the profound impact they had made on my life. Even though our time together was ending, we had forged the bonds of what I believed to be lifelong friendships.

Saying goodbye to everyone was hard. I had built such strong connections with my classmates and the staff at the academy that it was tough to leave. But I was headed home with a new vision for my life, and I was excited.

I was meticulously packing my belongings into my massive pink suitcase and preparing to bid farewell to the academy when a surge of emotions washed over me. The past two weeks had been a wild ride of getting uncomfortable, pushing my limits, grinding through challenges, and emerging victorious. I sat there in awe at how far I had come. The unassuming girl from

Canada, armed with nothing more than hope and a dream, had transformed into a certified firefighter, brimming with a newfound passion and purpose. A fire had been ignited within me that couldn't be put out. I was no longer content with merely pursuing the path of fire investigation. Fuck fire investigation altogether! I wanted to be a firefighter! But not just any firefighter. I aspired to shatter barriers and blaze a trail as the first female career firefighter in my hometown department!

I could envision it, and everything became vividly clear. Just because it had never been done before didn't mean it couldn't be done. With certainty, I knew I was going to be the one to do it!

Upon returning home, I wasted no time diving back into expanding my knowledge and enhancing my professional development. I was laser-focused on broadening my skill set and bolstering my resume by acquiring additional certifications. Months earlier, I had registered and paid for a spot in a fire investigation course, and I committed to completing the course like I had originally planned. Even though I was switching gears, I understood the value the course would bring to my scope of knowledge and my resume. The course location was logistically challenging—a twelve-hour drive—so I chose to fly and planned to stay at my friend's parents' home to ease the burden of accommodation expenses. His father was retired from the fire service, so I was thankful for their gracious invitation to stay with them and was eager to gain firsthand insight into the inner workings of life as a firefighter. I was also intrigued for the course and the opportunity to unravel the mysteries that may be concealed within the aftermath of a fire.

The classes proved to be both enriching and enlightening, unveiling a fascinating realm of knowledge. I found the subject matter very interesting. It did, however, confirm that fire investigation was not the career path I was destined for. My time there served as another valuable addition to my ever-expanding toolkit of skills and qualifications. I already stood out in my field, so it only seemed fitting to have additional training and certifications that could make me *really* stand out. **wink*

I remained committed to furthering my education and steadily chipped away at courses whenever time allowed. I was still balancing the demands of running my business and that alone was more than a full-time endeavor. It was all challenging but doable. I had created a list of necessary qualifications for a career in firefighting and my focus was directed at obtaining every single one. I acquired my airbrakes endorsement, which enabled me to operate firetrucks effectively, as well as my class 4 driver's license so I was positioned to drive an ambulance if needed. And finally, I invested in an industrial first aid certification. As taxing as it all was, I knew the time and effort invested in each qualification was bringing me one step closer to my dream. I was now fully equipped with the requisite credentials to put forward when the next job opening came available.

CHAPTER 4

I Have Never Felt So Small

After serving as an auxiliary firefighter for a couple of years, opportunities for permanent positions began to arise within the department. The first glimmer came in the form of a posting for a temporary six-month position, which was intended to fill the gap left by a member who was taking a leave of absence. A temporary position felt like the perfect chance to break into the department gently. I wasted no time in submitting my application and was ecstatic when I was chosen to take part in the hiring process.

A comprehensive physical test was first on the list. The assessment resembled an obstacle course and was designed to simulate various firefighting scenarios. Some of the tasks included extending and scaling a ladder, pulling hose lines, utilizing rescue tools, forcible entry simulation with a sledgehammer and tire, dragging a rescue manikin (dummy), etc. Another auxiliary member and I had been selected to undergo the rigorous examination, and it was being overseen by the deputy chief. We had just received a detailed demonstration of what lay ahead and were about to get started when, unexpectedly, two captains arrived to watch.

I was insanely nervous. I hadn't even geared up yet and my heart was pounding out of my chest and beads of sweat were forming. All of this was uncharted territory for me and the presence of an audience only intensified the pressure. I tried to remain confident, but their scrutinizing gazes made me question their intentions.

The other candidate had stepped up first to tackle the course, so I cheered him on and watched closely to gain any helpful insights for my own attempt. With a mix of anticipation and admiration, I watched as he navigated the challenges and completed the test with commendable proficiency. I offered him my congratulations and felt the pressure mount as I realized it was now my turn. I took a moment to steel my nerves, then donned the remainder of my gear. I was ready!

I focused on my breathing and navigated the obstacles quickly and efficiently. With each calculated step, I could feel their watchful eyes on me. Despite my best efforts to remain focused, the allure of stealing a glance in their direction was irresistible at times. Curiosity got the better of me. I glanced over at them only to witness their animated gestures and whispered conversation in full effect. That was a huge mistake on my part! Their presence, whether intended or not, was a potent distraction that sowed seeds of doubt within me and amplified my nerves.

I reached the point in the test where I had to drag the dummy across the truck bays, circumvent a cone, and return. I knew it was going to be difficult because they had chosen the heaviest one—close to 200lbs—which far surpassed my own weight. Yet I was confident I could handle it with the right technique. I squatted down low, grasped under its arms, and interlocked my hands across its chest. Holding it tight against my body, I took a deep breath and anchored my heels as I stood. Fuck, it was heavy! I had to drag it backward across the bay, so I maintained a keen eye to the side so I could gauge my distance and plot my turnaround. I fell into a rhythm, steadily progressing, when suddenly disaster struck. The heel of my boot snagged in a floor drain and sent me tumbling backward, falling flat on my back. The weight of the dummy crashed down hard on top of me. All the air was knocked out of my body. As I gasped, I heard a ring of laughter echo through the bays.

I lay there, utterly breathless, fighting desperately to hold back the flood of tears welling in my eyes. Through the blur of tears, I caught sight of a man walking toward me, his head shaking in amusement and a cruel snicker accompanying his every step. The humiliation was enough to break my fragile composure, and tears finally began streaming freely down my cheeks. As the captain drew nearer, still chuckling to himself, he leaned down and extended his hand in a mocking gesture of assistance.

"You're done!" he whispered.

I looked at him questioningly, searching for any hint of empathy, but his smile was dripping with malice, and his eyes were gleaming with wicked satisfaction.

He extended his hand a little farther because I hadn't taken his offer of assistance. His facade of concern was trying to mask the mockery in his eyes.

"Are you okay?" he asked, just loud enough for the gathering crowd to hear.

"No," I answered in a voice barely above a whisper.

The crowd of men had now encircled me. A few stepped forward to assist in removing the dummy off me and offer support as I struggled to gather myself up off the floor. Someone asked if I was okay, but I had no words and could only nod my head. I was not okay. Another person asked if I was going to continue, but I knew I couldn't muster the will. I still couldn't breathe from having the wind knocked out of me, and the weight of defeat and shame felt suffocating. I was so close to conquering the test, but every fiber of my being was screaming in protest. I knew I couldn't push forward. I was holding back intense emotions with a death grip and all I wanted was to get the fuck out of there and escape.

I held my composure the best I could as I doffed my gear and put it away. The deputy seemed disappointed for me and attempted to soften the blow of my defeat. I feigned resilience, brushed off the setback as a mere twist of fate, and insisted that I needed to leave because I was feeling unwell. He granted my release, and I made a beeline for the refuge of my truck, desperate to escape the prying eyes and stifling atmosphere.

In the truck, my whole body convulsed with the force of my sobs. I could barely breathe and began gasping for air. My head felt too heavy to hold as my forehead met the steering wheel for bracing. I was an absolute mess and desperate to get home. I frantically wiped the tears from my face, but I couldn't keep up with the steady flow.

"Breathe, Lynnette, just breathe!" I kept telling myself.

I needed to catch my breath, or I feared I would pass out. "Breathe, breathe, breathe," I chanted like a mantra. Slowly, I calmed down enough to drive, consumed by the overwhelming desire to flee to the comfort of home. Before I knew it, I found myself parked in the familiar embrace of my driveway, yet I had no recollection of driving there. My legs trembled beneath me as I staggered toward the house. I entered through the back door, closed it behind me, and collapsed. My entire body was wracked with weakness as waves of nausea washed over me. I sat hunched over with my head bowed to the floor in defeat, unable to move. I had never experienced such a depth of humiliation combined with overwhelming helplessness. My limbs felt like lead, my chest constricted with anguish, and every breath was a battle against the suffocating weight of despair. I didn't know what I was supposed to be doing, so I remained rooted to the spot with my mind and body frozen in a state of numbness. Moving seemed impossible. Honestly, I didn't even have the strength to try.

It felt like an eternity before I could muster enough strength to get off the floor. Each step was a painful effort as I held myself up with the railing and pushed my weary body to descend the stairs to my bedroom. I crawled onto the bed and collapsed in a heap of defeat. I pulled the blankets over me as I curled into fetal position. The tears resumed, cascading down my face and soaking my pillow. I remained there for hours, the weight of humiliation bearing down on me like a leaden blanket. My husband arrived and tried his best to console me, but I was not ready for comfort. Words felt like daggers, reminding me of my inadequacy. I just wanted to be left alone with my misery. After he left, I made a solemn vow to myself that I was done with firefighting and would renounce my role as an auxiliary first thing the next morning. The memory of my failure played on an endless loop in my mind and the thought of subjecting myself to such humiliation again was inconceivable. I couldn't fathom the purpose of attempting to persevere through such torment ever again. I couldn't and I wouldn't.

It was a nightmare playing out in real life. No matter how hard I tried, I couldn't shake the reverberations of that captain's evil laugh from my mind. He had made me feel small, insignificant, and powerless. The torment didn't end there. I continually subjected myself to the relentless punishment of replaying the scene over and over in my mind like a twisted movie reel. Every repetition only served to deepen the wounds as I scrutinized my failure. Doubt gnawed at me to the core as I questioned my abilities and my character and created fault of my own. How could I have let that happen? Why didn't I summon the strength to rise and finish what I had started? Why did I let him get to me?

One question remained unanswered: Why did he hate me so much? The mystery of his hatred was like a toxic cloud that poisoned every thought and cast a shadow on my sense of self-worth.

I was drowning in a tidal wave of humiliation and shame. Days passed in an agonizing blur and with each passing moment I sank deeper and deeper. I barely ate. I couldn't sleep. I had locked myself within the confines of my home and was a prisoner of my own thoughts. I had internalized it and mercilessly dissected every perceived flaw and failure. I became my own harshest critic, and my inner torment began spiraling out of control.

CHAPTER 5

Courage Under Fire

I was finally done grappling with my inner demons a few days later and summoned enough strength to emerge from the darkness. Exhausted, I pushed myself to stand once more. I had decided to confront my fears head-on and return to Tuesday night practice with my head held high. It took every ounce of courage I could muster to make myself walk through the front door. As I stepped into the firehall I was met with a spectrum of reactions. Some offered words of genuine support, and others gave an encouraging and optimistic, "Better luck next time." Their kindness soothed my wounded spirit. Of course, amidst the sea of support, one voice bit the air with heavy disappointment and disapproving remarks. But despite his doubt and disdain, I stood firm, determined to reclaim my sense of pride and prove that I was more than the sum of my failures.

Returning to the firehall was difficult and humbling. I hadn't wanted to do it, but I knew I needed to. The initial prospect filled me with dread and reluctance and waged an internal battle of conflicting voices that were both urging me to retreat and to press on. Even though I wanted desperately to surrender, the deep-rooted stubbornness within me refused. The road ahead loomed dauntingly because physical tests would still have to be taken, and many other challenges awaited. For the first time in my life, I questioned my abilities. Self-doubt was in the forefront and my confidence had been rocked. The sting of failure was deep and painful. Yet amidst the turmoil there was still a flicker of determination. I possessed an inner knowing that I couldn't ignore. I knew I had the physical prowess needed to successfully complete the obstacles. The real challenge for me was not my physical strength; it was in mastering the art of resilience in the face of scrutiny. That meant enduring the watchful eyes of others, enduring the judgment and opinions they threw around like parade candy. To be successful I would need to find a way to harness my inner power, silence the whispers of self-doubt, and stand tall in the face of adversity. Without a doubt, I knew I could do it.

I was feeling dissatisfied with the makeshift physical test at the firehall, so I approached the fire chief for his opinion on an alternative. I needed to prove to myself that I was capable so I could build up my confidence. But I needed to do it away from the firehall and any watchful eyes. After a candid conversation, he suggested a potential examination that took place in Edmonton, Alberta. I was intrigued by the prospect, so I delved into some research and felt that this new test just might provide the validation I was seeking. I would need to practice a few of the tasks presented in the test, so I reached out to a captain at the firehall who I was comfortable with and expressed my desire to hone my physical skills with some of the equipment. To my relief, he welcomed my request with open arms and offered his support and access to the equipment when he was on shift. For weeks, I immersed myself in training and seized every opportunity to familiarize myself with the tools and techniques that were required for my upcoming venture. With each practice run, my confidence grew, so I made the decision to take the plunge and book the test in Edmonton. Being a city that was six hours away presented a slight financial burden, as the transportation, accommodation, food, and registration were all at my own expense. I viewed it as a necessary investment in myself. I needed the chance to prove to both others and, more importantly, to myself that I could rise above the challenges that had once threatened to derail me. And so, with determination coursing through my veins, off to Edmonton I went!

The test was comprised of a series of grueling firefighting tasks and each one was timed individually to assess my proficiency under pressure. I had dedicated numerous hours to practice and preparation, so I was approaching it with a quiet confidence and a deep knowing that I had what it took to succeed. I was given a quick briefing of rules and expectations at each station and then got right to it. As the test unfolded, I tackled each task methodically as the examiner stood watch with his clipboard and stopwatch. Task by task, I pressed forward and summoned every ounce of strength and skill at my disposal. With the weight of the gear bearing down on me, and the intensity mounting at every station, I was pushed to exhaustion. Finally, it was over. I had completed every task, and a swell of pride washed over me.

It was the moment of reckoning as I sat down with the examiner to review my test results. As he methodically went through the checklist one by one, my heart raced with anticipation and excitement.

"Pass, pass, pass." His words reverberated through my mind like a chorus of victory. "Fail, pass, pass, pass."

But that one word hit me like a sudden thunderclap. *Fail? What?* How could that be? I was completely shocked! The examiner explained the reason for the failure; one of the tasks was a mere two seconds shy of the mark. *Two fucking seconds!* I was in complete disbelief.

"Two seconds?" I had to say it out loud to myself to comprehend it.

I questioned him repeatedly, hoping against hope for a different outcome, but the verdict remained unchanged. In that moment, the world seemed to crumble around me. The sense of devastation was all too familiar as hot and bitter tears welled in my eyes. I had poured everything I had into every task, and here I was with the reality of failure once again. My heart sank. I left the facility with my head down and climbed into the truck. The tears flowed rapidly, and they didn't subside for the entire six-hour journey home. I was mentally, emotionally, and physically exhausted. The weight of failure was once again too much to bear.

It took me several days to gather the courage and compose myself enough to return to the firehall and face the fire chief with my test results. With a heavy heart and a knot of apprehension in my stomach, I braced myself for the uncomfortable conversation. To my surprise, his response was unexpectedly comforting. With genuine empathy he reassured me that missing the mark by a mere two seconds did not diminish my abilities in his eyes. His words of encouragement offered a much-needed respite from my relentless self-criticism about being a failure. He asked permission to share my results with the union representatives and see if they would be considered adequate for the next hiring round. But despite his efforts, the outcome was exactly what I had expected: a resounding no. I was disappointed yet understood their reasoning behind the decision. I didn't pass, and in the world of firefighting, there was no room for failing to meet the standard, no matter how slight. The weight of that missed opportunity hung heavily over me and was a constant reminder of my perceived shortcomings. Missing one task by two seconds was beyond infuriating and did nothing but fuel the flames of self-doubt and self-criticism.

To my surprise, not a single soul broached the subject or tried to use it against me. The conspicuous absence of any mention of my setback felt eerie and fucked with my head a little. It was as if a veil of secrecy had been drawn over the topic and it left me to wonder what was really simmering behind the scenes. In a twisted way, I had already grown to expect the jabs and the belittling comments. But this time was different. Taunts and jeers were replaced with an unsettling silence. At least, to my face. In a way, the silence was more deafening than any insult could've been. It was disconcerting but at the same time a welcome reprieve.

I felt increasingly irritated at the dilemma of what steps to take next. All because of one looming challenge. Passing a physical test! I had a whirlwind of questions spinning in my mind. Should I invest more money to retake the test? Was it even endorsed by fire departments? Or was there another option out there? Just as I was mulling over my options, the department made the decision for me. They had decided that the Candidate Physical Ability Test (CPAT) would now be the mandatory benchmark for their new recruits. Curious, I delved into some research and discovered a troubling trend: the CPAT was notorious for being particularly difficult for women. According to various articles I stumbled upon, a staggering 97 percent of female candidates failed to make the cut on their first two attempts, leaving only one more chance. The timing of their mandate felt perfectly pointed considering the upcoming full-time positions they knew I was going to be applying for. That added some unwelcome pressure for sure. But I couldn't dwell on their potential ulterior motives, and succumbing to self-doubt was a luxury I couldn't afford. My focus needed to shift squarely onto the CPAT—and pronto! It was time to roll up my sleeves and get to work on some serious training.

After thoroughly dissecting the test course online, I crafted myself a training regimen that was tailored to its unique demands. I invested in a weighted vest and a trove of additional weights because I needed it to mirror the exact load I would have to bear during the test. I had to get creative and sought out unconventional training venues—from playgrounds to steep hills, the confines of the gym, and equipment at the firehall like I had done previously. Of course, there were elements of the test that defied replication without elaborate setups, such as constructing a large blacked-out tunnel with entanglement props and obstacles inside. Instead, I embraced the challenge and improvised the best I could. The test itself demanded the completion of eight distinct events in a seamless, continuous flow within a tight time frame of ten minutes and twenty seconds. Was it terrifying? Undoubtedly. Was it achievable? *Fuck yes!*

The closest test site to me was Calgary, Alberta, which was a grueling nine-hour trek by car. Determination was fueling my every move, and I needed to act on it. I secured a test date and only divulged my plans to my family. I was very deliberate in shielding myself from any external pressures because it was pivotal that this quest be free of any distractions or discouragement. This journey was about reclaiming my sense of self-worth and represented a personal odyssey toward redemption. My past failures still weighed heavily on my shoulders and had tanked my confidence and self-esteem. This wasn't just about passing a test; it was about reclaiming my narrative and proving to myself that I was capable and possessed the grit to make it happen.

Every aspect of this endeavor—the test itself, the travel arrangements, the accommodations, the time away from my business—came at a steep personal cost. It was a financial burden, but every penny spent was a necessary sacrifice for my aspirations. I was investing in my future and laying the steppingstones on the path toward fulfilling my dream of becoming a firefighter.

Embarking on this quest felt daunting as fuck, and I didn't want to go it alone. So, I enlisted the one person I knew whose presence of grit and strength would push me harder than ever: my father. His blend of tough love and unwavering belief in my abilities would provide me the confidence to face the challenge. But unknowingly I was doing it for both of us—driven not only by my relentless drive to succeed, but by the need to make him proud.

The testing location required an entire day of travel and was scheduled for the following morning. As we arrived at the facility, I was met by the evaluator, who couldn't help but express curiosity for me doing the test on my own. I shared a glimpse of my journey and story with him, and the reasons why I was there. His surprise was apparent, but his response was very encouraging. He took us down into the testing space and gave a detailed description of each event and what would determine an automatic failure. I asked a few questions for clarification, then he gave me a few moments of solitude to gather my thoughts and mentally steel myself for the test. Alone in the room, I gave myself a serious pep talk of empowerment and courage as I paced back and forth. I took a couple of deep breaths and signaled to him that I was ready. My nerves were coursing through me like an electric current, and I planned to use them to propel me forward. I entered the floor with fierce confidence and vowed to drain every ounce of effort out there on the course. I put on the weighted vest and stepped up onto the step mill. Three, two, one . . . go!

As I made my way through each event, the evaluator stood vigilant to ensure I was meticulously completing each task. I noted the stopwatch in his hand as that tiny piece of equipment held my fate. A backup timer stood poised in the distance. I could hear the echoes of my father's cheers and, when needed, I would glance over at him for his reassuring nod. I was approaching the final event and hadn't been stopped for any infractions or time expiration, so I dug deep and summoned every last bit of strength I could muster. The crescendo was a demanding ceiling push/pull that counted reps, and each one happened faster and harder than the last. Done! I looked at the evaluator, who wore a jubilant grin and as he turned the stopwatch to reveal the results of my efforts. He told me that I had done it in under ten minutes! I had completed it with time to spare!

I collapsed to my knees and was overcome with emotion. Tears freely streamed down my cheeks, escaping from a place of inner knowing. They were a much-needed release of self-doubt and a reclamation of the power I had lost. Deep within, I always knew I could do it, but I needed a fair opportunity and a safe space to try. I was exhausted but exhilarated and reveled in the moment as a rush of pride washed over me. The fatigue was mental, and the sweat was physical. I looked up as my father approached—the smile on his face said it all—he was proud. He held out his hand and I reached for it, allowing him to help me off the floor. As I stood, he embraced me in a firm hug, and I could feel the intensity of his emotions, a mix of joy and pride that matched my own. I was on cloud nine and couldn't wipe the well-earned smile off my face as we departed the facility.

Before the test, my nerves had robbed me of my appetite. But now, with success in hand, we were going to celebrate with a satisfying lunch. I clutched my hard-earned certificate as I entered the restaurant, filled with a deep satisfaction and sense of triumph that I was unable to resist admiring it. I fucking did it! Against the odds, I did it, and it was everything I had hoped for and more.

Our lunch conversation revolved entirely around the test and the sweet victory of passing it. We laughed about how my success would undoubtedly piss off the people who wished for me to fail, and the satisfaction that brought me was undeniable. My father shared in that joy—his pride mirroring my own—as we both savored the moment. It was confirmation that bringing him along had been the right choice.

I returned home with a regained sense of a confidence that filled a void that had been empty for far too long. It was a welcome sensation and one I welcomed wholeheartedly. Naturally, my first destination was the firehall because I couldn't wait to share my achievement. As I stepped into the building, I was greeted by a firefighter and a captain whose expressions revealed they were less than excited to see me. Undeterred, I inquired about the fire chief's availability to see me, and they wanted to know the intention of my visit. I noticed their curious glances toward the certificate I was clutching. With a smile, I nonchalantly announced that I had passed the CPAT and wanted to give him a copy of my certificate and proudly held it out for them to see. Their reactions were not what I had anticipated. Instead of congratulations, there was a serious lack of enthusiasm and appeared to be a mixture of surprise and resentment.

"How many times before you passed?" the captain immediately fired off.

"One," I responded, aware of his skepticism.

"Yeah, right," the captain muttered under his breath as he rolled his eyes and walked away.

I was left standing with the firefighter so I asked him if he could please check on the fire chief's availability. After a brief wait, he motioned for me to proceed to the office at the end of the hall. I entered and proudly handed him my certificate. His genuine happiness for my accomplishment was evident as he gave me a firm handshake and a sincere congratulations. I instantly felt the sense of validation and recognition I had desperately needed.

As anticipated, I encountered some pushback but was quite taken aback when I discovered that accusations were flying about the authenticity of my claim regarding the number of attempts I'd made at the test. A couple of the men stood so certain in my supposed falsehoods that they insisted on seeking verification on my statement with the test authorities in Calgary. I found their disbelief puzzling as I wasn't sure why the number of attempts mattered, but I encouraged them to seek the verification if they felt it necessary. The outcome of their purported investigation never surfaced. I received conflicting reports that they had followed through on their threat and was also told that they had not. I had my suspicions but decided to leave things alone. Either way, the fact remained the same: I had triumphed over the CPAT on my first attempt.

CHAPTER 6

A Trust Test: The Chief's Word

Fast-forward one year to the beginning of summer 2009. The fire department announced a coveted opening for a full-time position. I had been anticipating this, so I promptly submitted my application package. Shortly thereafter, I received the gratifying news that I had been shortlisted and was invited for an interview. A large panel interview was a completely new experience for me and required diligent preparation. I was armed with an interview guidebook and had received some valuable insights from my fire academy friends who had already navigated similar interviews successfully. Although the specific interview questions were a mystery, I felt reassured and confident by my preparation and my support network. The interview panel was comprised of an array of fire department and City Hall personnel, along with one member from the union executive. I met each question with a poised response and exited the interview feeling just as confident as I had going in. Now all that remained was the anticipatory wait for that definitive call. *The* call to confirm I was the chosen candidate.

I was caught off guard as the fire chief's number flashed on my phone screen while working at the hair salon. I paused and stared at the phone for a moment, my heart pounding with anticipation. I calmly answered the call with professional composure. Excitement was bubbling within me, but I maintained a calm exterior as I listened carefully. I expected to hear words of congratulations and an offer of the coveted position; instead, my smile faded as the fire chief stated he needed to speak with me and requested a face-to-face meeting. He asked if we could meet in a neutral location away from prying ears. Although perplexed by this unexpected turn of events, I agreed to meet in a donut shop parking lot later that afternoon. After hanging up the phone, I stood there for a moment, pondering the purpose of the meeting. I couldn't help but be intrigued, yet I was also curious and confused.

Struggling to focus amidst the hum of the salon, I was constantly glancing at the clock and willing time to move faster. It truly felt like time was standing still. My mind was looping through all the possible reasons for the impending meeting. Initially, I entertained the possibility that it was a simple congratulatory gesture, but the notion was swiftly dismissed as illogical. Such a gesture wouldn't necessitate all this secrecy, away from the prying ears of the firehall. That part of the puzzle was odd and left me at a loss. I was frustrated by my inability to decipher the chief's intentions and had to accept that patience was my only option. However, patience was never my strong suit, and the agonizing wait felt like torture. As I wrapped up with my final client, I abandoned any pretense of tidying up and left behind a mess that I would come back to clean later.

It was a very short drive from my salon to the donut shop, but I seemed to encounter every slow driving farmer along the way. As I approached the meeting destination, I looked in my rearview mirror and discovered the fire chief's vehicle trailing close behind me. Seeing him there intensified the pounding of my heart. We maneuvered into the parking lot one after the other, then into parking spaces side by side. I took a few deep breaths to steady my nerves before I stepped out of my truck. He was already standing at the back of his, so I straightened my posture and walked over and shook his hand to say hello. It was clear by his facial expression and his body language that something of significance was about to go down. He started by expressing gratitude for my willingness to meet, then somberly acknowledged he had a very difficult decision he was facing and needed me to hear him out. He had my full attention, and I listened intently as he began to outline the situation.

The successful candidate for the upcoming position would be integrated into the crew led by the very captain who had openly expressed his dislike for me and had caused me considerable distress in the past. My heart sank as I nodded in understanding. It was not the news I had hoped for, but I kept an open mind as he continued to explain the circumstances. With a commendable display of honesty and integrity, the chief acknowledged that morally he couldn't put me on that crew. He knew my earnest desire for the position and recognized, rightfully, that my qualifications should grant it to me. Ethically, though, he was obligated to prioritize not only my well-being but that of the department as well.

"I need you to trust me," the chief stated, looking me straight in the eyes.

With a solemn tone, he revealed a glimmer of hope amidst the disappointment. There was going to be another position coming available in a couple of months that would be under the leadership of a captain who not only accepted me but also respected me. It was an assurance of a safer and more supportive environment, and that prospect resonated with both of us. I expressed my sincere appreciation and gratitude for his honesty and genuine concern for my well-being. I admitted that the news had fallen short of my initial hopes, but I completely accepted and understood his rationale.

As I drove away from our discussion, I was filled with a mixture of disappointment, frustration, and confidence. I was disappointed that I had to wait, and extremely frustrated that it was because of someone else's lack of tact and integrity. But I felt confident that I could trust in the chief's plan and for him to follow through on the next position. Despite our limited acquaintance, he had only shown me consistent integrity, which had established a strong sense of trust. In fact, I had just gained immense respect for him as a man and as a capable leader.

As anticipated, another candidate was hired for the position. I'd be lying if I said it didn't bother me. It stung. But I had reconciled with the outcome and knew deep down that it was for the greater good of all involved. I had a genuine aversion to working under the captain of that crew. I also believe, without a shadow of a doubt, that had we been paired together, the department would have been in jeopardy, and one of us likely would've ended up in jail.

CHAPTER 7

Betrayal Behind Closed Doors

Life carried on in a steady rhythm for me as I waited patiently for the next position to come open. I was managing my salon business, faithfully attending Tuesday night practices, and responding to calls of duty whenever I was paged out. I had the opportunity to apply my skills and training on several large and challenging fires. One of the most memorable was a grain elevator fire, which required precise coordination and teamwork due to the size and complexity of the structure. Another involved a massive warehouse fire, where we not only battled the blaze but the extreme heat conditions. I was also tasked with responding to an additional call that day, putting on an air pack (SCBA) and conducting an interior search with fire extinguishment on a mobile home. In each situation, I was able to demonstrate my capabilities in such high stakes scenarios and contribute to the team's success.

I was contacted one day out of the blue by a member at the department and told there were undisclosed developments that he felt may need my attention. Naturally, my curiosity was piqued. I was then grossly informed that there were private backroom discussions taking place within the confines of the firehall, and they were being orchestrated by certain members with the explicit aim of brainstorming ways to stop me from getting hired.

By that time, I had cultivated a small circle of "friends" who were playing both ends from the middle. They were not in favor of the shit that was going on and were willing to share insider insights whenever I inquired, but they also felt bound by the brotherhood. Their loyalty to their brothers often conflicted with their personal beliefs. For me, however, the source of information mattered less than the information itself. This juicy piece of information, however, was recounted from more than one individual who had experienced the situation firsthand from behind closed doors. It was intriguingly corroborated by another man who, despite being part of the brotherhood, had found himself mysteriously excluded from the inner circle altogether.

I struggled to wrap my head around this situation. I had never encountered this type of behavior before. I worked in the beauty industry where salon spaces were always portrayed as a place for women to gossip and spread rumors. But this scenario involved only men, and the dynamics were far more toxic. I envisioned high school bullying tactics to be similar to what these men were doing; where individuals would band together to exert power and try to intimidate others into conformity.

I was utterly shocked by the disturbing details that were shared with me about these meetings. It was alarming to learn that lies were being fabricated and exaggerated about me, as they were searching for any shred of information they could get to use against me. What disturbed me even more was the active involvement of certain individuals who were willingly engaging in this deceitful plotting. I was told that the atmosphere in some of the meetings was highly charged as certain individuals were resorting to aggressive tactics, including yelling and making threats toward those who dared to challenge the plan or didn't agree to take part in it.

This behavior was so hard for me to comprehend, and my mind was a whirlwind of perplexing questions. Why did they feel compelled to launch such a relentless campaign to discredit me? Why did they hate me so much? For days, I carefully sifted through my memories and dissected every past interaction with everyone involved. It was like going through old movie reels. I replayed conversations, I scrutinized actions, and I analyzed body language. I couldn't grasp what I was missing so I turned the spotlight on myself. I started questioning whether I had inadvertently said or done something offensive. I agonized over whether my demeanor had ever come across as bitchy or unkind. I subjected myself to relentless self-examination and dissected my own behaviors for any hint of wrongdoing or a potential misstep that could have triggered their hostility. I picked every piece of myself apart and still couldn't identify anything significant enough to warrant the intensity of their actions against me.

A storm of emotions engulfed me. I was angry, I was deeply hurt, and I was sad. The anger was for the injustice of the situation. The hurt was because my trust had been betrayed, and my efforts were disregarded. Beneath it all was a deep well of sadness that stemmed from the realization that even though I had shown unwavering dedication over the past four years, I was being unjustly targeted.

I prided myself on being a team player, working hard, and being one of first ones to arrive and the last ones to leave. I always aimed to be supportive, positive, and encouraging to others. My commitment extended to attentively listening to direction and dutifully following orders. I was always eager to contribute in any way possible. I looked at it from every conceivable angle, and it didn't make sense to me. So I did the only thing I knew how to do with what I had been told. I internalized the accusations and criticisms that were hurled my way and owned them as if they were my own.

It didn't help matters that I was in the beginning stages of separation with my husband, which magnified my feelings of insecurity. I knew we shouldn't have gotten married to begin with—even our counsellor had warned against it—but I had clung to a fragile hope that our relationship could defy the odds. Perhaps I could prove everyone wrong. Through marriage I hoped to validate my own worth and prove to myself that I was worthy of love. Now here I was, admitting defeat in my marriage and facing the stark reality that it was flawed from inception. Whether it was the lack of approval from my father, the dissolution of my marriage, or the scrutiny of the men at the firehall, I felt defined by my shortcomings and found myself turning up the volume on proving my worth. I hadn't been able to prove it in my childhood or my marriage, so now the direction of my focus was on the firehall. I was a strong, capable, independent woman, and I would show *all* of them that I would do everything I was told I couldn't. I was on a mission to prove to them that I was worthy.

CHAPTER 8

There Are Strings Attached

I got *the* call. I was in between appointments, sitting at the front desk in my salon, when my phone buzzed, flashing the fire chief's name across the screen. It felt like total déjà vu. I paused for a moment to compose a calm and professional demeanor before answering. I greeted him and then listened as he told me he was delivering long-awaited good news. I was the successful candidate, and he was happily offering me the full-time firefighter position. *Eeeeeeekkk!* I happily accepted his offer and was filled with immense excitement and relief. Complete full-body excitement for getting the job, and deep relief because he had kept his word and followed through from our conversation a few months prior.

I made a flurry of phone calls to share my exhilarating news and then snapped back to reality to survey my surroundings. I had a lot of organizing, planning, and figuring out to do. I was operating an extremely busy spa alongside two other women while also maintaining a substantial hair clientele. I was mentally prepared that when I got the job, I would transition my business into a room in my basement at home, so I could continue to do hair on my days off from the fire department. The career change meant a significant financial setback, so I would need to offset that by juggling both jobs for an unforeseeable amount of time. The career move brought benefits that being a sole proprietor didn't have, such as paid holidays, medical benefits, and a pension. However, those things didn't compensate for the severe loss to my income stream, so I would be necessitating sacrifices to maintain equilibrium. Ultimately, I was embarking on a new career path I was extremely passionate about, which overshadowed the challenges. With time and effort, I would find my footing and thrive.

Things were moving at a rapid pace. Two days later I met with the fire chief and union rep to go over the intricacies of imminent hire. Unfortunately, my excitement was swiftly tempered by unexpected conditions attached to my employment. It was revealed that they deemed my CPAT certificate invalid due to its expiration five months prior—even though it was valid when I applied for the position and interviewed. As a result, they were requiring me to complete the test *again* before the conclusion of my six-month probationary period. What struck me the hardest was the realization that this decision wasn't driven from management; it was being influenced by the union. The very brotherhood I was poised to become a sister in.

The one-year expiration date on my certificate had never been understood to align with the standards set by the entity administering the CPAT. After all, the document prominently bore the insignia of that fire department across the top. Until now, there had never been any indication that our department was adopting the same stringent regulations. But since I was the first individual in the department to have undergone the CPAT process, it only seemed fitting that they were establishing rules on the fly to accommodate their needs.

I had no words. I released a slow and measured exhale, the stirrings of anger simmering within me. Negative thoughts began to infiltrate my mind, and my frustration was intensifying.

Are you fucking kidding me? my inner monologue repeatedly questioned.

Beneath the table my hands were on my lap, my fingers intertwined, and I was tightly squeezing them together to keep that voice muzzled on the inside. I refused to show them any signs of the emotional turmoil raging within me. I wasn't giving them the satisfaction of witnessing my distress. I concealed it behind a facade of smiles and pretended that their actions were inconsequential. I was happy to go along with their game. Even though I was dying inside, I recognized their maneuvers for what they were: another attempt to assert dominance and maintain a power position.

I had to get myself in check. Regardless of the looming challenge ahead, I reminded myself that I had a six-month window to navigate through the complexities. Dwelling on it right now would only discourage me and dampen the joy I deserved to feel. I had worked my ass off, waited my turn, and was finally hired for the job I wanted. It was time to revel in this monumental achievement. I deserved to celebrate, and celebrate I would! I allowed myself to bask in the glory that I was writing an exciting new chapter in my life, and there was no way in hell I was going to allow "the boys' club" to steal it.

Over the next week, my schedule was a whirlwind as I shuttled between the firehall, my home, and the salon. At the firehall I underwent fittings for my uniforms and received the essential gear I would need to start my new job. Back at home I was knee-deep in salon renovations and meticulously orchestrating every detail in hopes of a seamless shift from the spa location to my home-based business. Even with the time constraints, I had a sense of reassurance that was born from the methodical preparation I had done. All my clients had been made aware in advance of my impending career change and had remained loyal and solid by my side. They had tagged along for the entire ride thus far and provided me with stability and reassurance amidst the flurry of changes. I loved them with my whole heart, and their presence was a constant source of comfort. Their encouragement and support meant the world to me, and I was beyond grateful for the bond we shared. I found security in knowing that I was still going to be doing their hair and spending time with them. I needed them through this transition and loved them for enduring it with me.

I was now in the middle of the separation with my husband. So far, we had managed to maintain a veil of privacy around our situation. I was starting my new career that involved only men, and I knew how the news of leaving my husband would spread rumors like wildfire. I had been asked many times what my husband thought of me being surrounded by men, and I assured them it wasn't an issue. A few professed their opinions that a real man would never allow his wife to work with only men, but I just ignored them. I wasn't prepared to confront them head-on just yet and decided to cross that bridge when I came to it. I remained focused on both my salon relocation and launching into my new professional chapter. Thankfully my soon-to-be-ex-husband proved to be very understanding, which allowed us to navigate our separation with grace and dignity. Despite the dissolution of our romantic relationship, we had cultivated a solid friendship, which was one of the main reasons for our separation. Ours was not a tale of bitterness or anything nasty; it was merely that we functioned better as friends than spouses, and we both recognized it. Our amicable rapport shielded us from prying eyes and unwarranted scrutiny. By remaining cordial and civil, we were able to keep our personal affairs out of the public eye. The timing for this transition was far from ideal for me, but it just meant I was venturing into a completely new life.

With efficiency and organization being two special qualities of mine, I had every detail attended to and every item ticked off my checklist. Everything was perfectly prepared for the dawn of my inaugural day as a firefighter.

CHAPTER 9

You're On Your Own

The day had finally arrived! Anticipation had been building for what felt like an eternity. As expected, sleep had eluded me the night before due to my excitement. I rose early and did a light workout to try and soothe my nerves. I felt invigorated and prepared to tackle my first day as a career firefighter. This was an historic day, not just for me, but for the entire department. I had been hired as *the* first ever career female firefighter at Dawson Creek Fire Rescue.

The night before I had thoroughly prepared for my trailblazing debut. Every detail had been meticulously attended to. From packing my lunch and snacks, to pressing my uniform—yes, I ironed it!—to envisioning myself putting it on a hundred times. I had never worn a uniform before. To me, it represented significant responsibility. This wasn't a dress rehearsal, and the appointed hour was rapidly approaching.

Standing in front of the mirror, I thoughtfully dressed myself in the crisp navy-blue uniform and savored the sensation of every button, zip, and tuck. Even though it was tailored for a man's frame and didn't fit me properly, I would still wear it with pride. I stared at my reflection in the mirror, outlined by the crisp lines of the uniform. I couldn't help but feel a profound shift within me as I embodied my newfound identity with purpose, responsibility, and duty. I affixed my name tag to the top of my right breast pocket and smiled as my finger traced over the word *firefighter* engraved beneath my name. It was more than just a name tag; it was a hard-earned badge of honor. The package was complete. I was ready to go—with time to spare. I found myself pacing anxiously and kept watch as the hands on the clock ticked at a snail's pace.

I could hardly contain my excitement to start my day at the firehall. Living in such close proximity meant that the commute was a mere two minutes. I pulled into a parking spot and allowed myself a few extra moments inside my truck to collect my thoughts and absorb the magnitude of my career decision. My heart felt like it was going to pound right through my chest.

As I stepped into the firehall, I immediately became engulfed in an atmosphere that radiated tension and filled me with discomfort like I had never experienced before, which said a lot given everything I had already been through. Despite regularly attending Tuesday night practices and actively participating in calls over the past four years, the space now felt foreign and unwelcoming. The air felt thick and heavy, and it was hard for me to breathe; the atmosphere had transformed and become dense and suffocating. While most of my coworkers' faces bore expressions of polite acknowledgment, there were a select few whose dislike for my presence was unmistakable. Their silent hostility simmered beneath the surface, and their resentment was evident in their hard stares.

The day kicked off with a series of meetings. First was a session with management where we delved into a mountain of paperwork. From there, I made my way to City Hall for a session with the HR department, filling out a sea of forms and documents. In between the administrative tasks, I connected with the on-duty crew for coffee breaks and lunch. As a probationary firefighter (probie) there was a huge learning curve to the culture, the intricacies of the fire service hierarchy, and the inner workings of our station. There was a wealth of behind-the-scenes operations that I never got to observe as an auxiliary. One thing I knew for certain was that knowing and mastering my role was paramount. I was armed with a notepad and absorbed every insight like a sponge, diligently recording every tidbit of information that was being passed onto me, as well as anything I thought might be crucial for my development. As I observed the seasoned firefighters fielding phone calls, I took detailed mental and physical notes on what they said and did. Due to my coffee aversion, I had to learn the art of brewing coffee; my lack of skill drew some serious digs. I had never drunk coffee, couldn't even stand the smell of it, so I never saw a need to know how to make it. Well, that was about to change because coffee in the fire station was a staple, and it was the probie's job to not only make sure that a pot was always brewed, but to serve it as well. Thankfully, I was a quick study on the coffee culture! Any opportunity I got throughout the day to shadow my colleagues, I soaked in their expertise and jotted down pages and pages of notes—everything from dispatch protocols to making a perfect pot of coffee.

Later that afternoon the on-duty captain beckoned me into the dispatch room so we could "have a chat." He slid the window shut and closed the door behind us, motioning for me to take a seat. Then he settled into a chair opposite mine, wearing a stone-faced expression as he fixed his gaze upon me.

"You did it. You must be so excited," he said. "This must be the most exciting day of your life."

"Yes, it is," I responded with a wary smile, wondering what was coming next.

"Well, there's something you need to know," he said with an air of nonchalance. "We've all talked, and we're all in agreement that if you get yourself into any kind of trouble, we're not coming to save you." With chilling clarity, he looked me dead in the eye and added a final blow. "You're on your own."

I couldn't move. I sat there, frozen, as if time itself had ground to a halt. I could feel the blood draining from my face and the air leaving my lungs without the promise of returning. My gaze fixated on his lips; they were still moving in a steady rhythm, but I couldn't hear any sound. I was lost in the deafening roar of my own apprehension and his suffocating grip of intimidation. Through the haze of panic, I heard him ask me if I understood, and all I could muster was a feeble smile and a slight nod of my head. I was in complete disbelief and didn't understand why he basically told me no one had my back, and they would leave me to die! I felt utterly powerless and consumed with confusion at being cornered by his threat. As quickly as this new chapter had started, all the joy and pride I'd felt had extinguished.

He rose from his seat. With weak legs I followed his lead and stood up. He extended his hand for a handshake, and I forced my trembling hand to meet his grasp halfway. I prayed he couldn't feel the tremors. He offered a hollow "congratulations" before releasing my hand with a forced smile. I had seen that smile before, and the evil behind it sent shivers down my spine. He walked out of the dispatch room with an air of casual indifference, and I remained rooted in position, struggling to move. I slowly reopened the sliding window, trying to buy myself some time before having to face the others in the firehall. I felt as if I had just had the wind knocked out of me and couldn't stand up straight. I leaned heavily onto the desk with both hands and tried to steady myself. I took slow breaths, trying to get some air back into my lungs and reclaim some semblance of composure. I had the rest of the day yet to finish and had no idea how the fuck that was going to happen.

I immersed myself in tasks and tried to fill every moment with activity, but I was having a really hard time concentrating. No matter how hard I tried, I couldn't stop the relentless echo of his ruthless words. With every repetition, my heart would thunder against my chest like a drumbeat, and I would have to stop what I was doing and try to breathe. I couldn't seem to get enough air and felt like I was suffocating.

I struggled with the harsh reality that not only was I an outsider in the department, but I was also an outcast. I had hoped to gain a few friends among my peers, but I honestly didn't know if I would. I knew there had been private, back-room meetings with the members who tried to sabotage my efforts at getting hired, but had they really collaborated on the decision to leave me on my own if I was in trouble? Firefighters depend heavily on teamwork, trust, and clearheaded leadership. Yet this captain was willing to jeopardize my life with an act that was blatantly dangerous and irresponsible. The betrayal cut deep, and fear gripped me with an icy hand. I felt alone and very vulnerable, which broke my heart and scared the shit out of me at the same time. The brotherhood I had aspired to join had just revealed depths of darkness far greater than I had ever imagined. I honestly didn't know the scope of what or who I was truly dealing with.

That conversation changed me and the way I would do my job. I just didn't know it yet.

The first eight weeks my schedule was dedicated to familiarization and intensive training. Working consecutive day shifts from Monday through Thursday afforded me the opportunity to interact with all the different crews as they cycled through their rotations. This allowed me to become acquainted with the unique dynamics of each team while immersing myself in the intricacies of our dispatch protocols. We were the designated 911 fire dispatch center for the South Peace region and our responsibilities extended far beyond simply answering emergency phone calls. Each call brought with it a cascade of critical decisions, from assessing the nature and severity of the situation to dispatching the appropriate resources in a timely manner. With each ring of the dreadful stinger—the volume and sound of it could give you a heart attack—I learned the art of navigating a labyrinth of questions to ask, procedures and protocols to follow, followed by coordinating firefighters and other emergency services to respond effectively. Multiple lines were often ringing at once as I paged firefighters, performed radio communications with responding units, and scribed detailed notes for the reports. There was a lot to learn!

Having the opportunity to work alongside all the crews was a fascinating experience. Each captain was distinctly unique, and their leadership styles varied significantly. There were four completely different personalities, rules, expectations, and each with their own way of doing things. I had the difficult job of navigating through these diverse environments and needed to constantly adapt and morph into different versions of myself depending on whose command I was under. Some days I was welcomed with open arms, treated with respect, and given equal opportunity to learn and grow. Other days I was belittled and treated like a complete inconvenience.

"You're a nice enough girl. I like you," I was told. "But you don't belong here. And in case you haven't noticed, we don't *want* you here."

The remaining days I was to be seen and not heard. I was expected to blend into the background as if I were invisible. Every two days I needed to alter my persona, and I quickly learned which role I was to play dependent on whose presence I was in.

I deeply appreciated the individuals who accepted me and treated me with fairness during my initiation phase. I was grateful for their patience and integrity, as I acquired so many invaluable lessons from them. In an environment that was often marked by hostility, I cherished every interaction with the calm and understanding individuals, who not only offered guidance but offered moments of playfulness as well. They played occasional pranks and hazing rituals on me. They set up a trip wire rigged to a paintball gun that was filled with flour. They doused me with buckets of water in the hose tower. They locked me in the boiler room by removing the inside door handle, then simulated an emergency call by setting off the stinger and pretending to respond without me. Yes, they were pranks or acts of hazing, but they gave me a sense of belonging. They were integral to the culture and made me feel included.

After a few weeks, I found myself back among the original crew I had started with. The on-duty captain decided to initiate some SCBA drills throughout the firehall, specifically designed for me and the colleague who was hired before me. Attentively, I listened to his instructions, got into my gear as calmly as I could muster, and then donned my SCBA. I worked my way through the obstacles he laid out for us and followed his directions on what to do next. He had us crawling under trucks, scaling stairs, toggling our air supply, and then finishing by dragging a rescue dummy through the bays around the parked trucks. It became very evident early on that the captain had set up a subtle competition between my colleague and me, with his favor obviously leaning toward the other individual. He was constantly encouraging him and praising his skill, as well as highlighting his achievements, and suggesting I emulate his performance. There were two other guys on the crew, and one of them joined us at the beginning, but the captain quickly told him he didn't need to take part. The other one just observed as it all unfolded, and the other soon joined him. I wondered if perhaps they were finding as much amusement in it as the captain was. He wore a self-satisfied grin and laughed to himself in between bellowing out orders on what we were to do next. He had us run through numerous rounds and variations of the drill.

It was now time to break for lunch. We were instructed to remove our gear and refill our air cylinders before heading upstairs to eat. After ensuring everything was back in ready working order, we ascended to the day room where everyone was already wrapping up their meals. I grabbed my lunch from the fridge, quietly settled at the table, and listened to the conversations swirling around me as I ate.

I was still eating when the captain's booming voice suddenly hollered out, "Sixty seconds!"

That meant we had sixty seconds to get into our gear, so we instantly abandoned our meals and sprinted downstairs. As swiftly as I could, I geared up and donned my SCBA. The captain had followed us down and voiced the directions of a new drill. He wanted us on air, but we were to remove the backpack, slide under a narrow gap beneath the bay door, push the pack out in front of us, and then repeat the process. Once we got back

inside, we put our packs back on and then shuttled up and down the stairs carrying various tools or hose rolls. With every pass I tried to avoid the captain's gaze but would catch the occasional glimpse through the side of my mask. His expression revealed that the gears were turning in his mind, and I was curious what was coming next. As our final lap around the stairs concluded, he opened the bay door and directed us to drag the dummy from the hose tower, through the truck bays, and then out to the end of the ramp and back.

I was instantly reminded of my earlier fiasco with dragging the dummy during my first physical test, and it felt like this directive was a deliberate effort to recreate the circumstances of that fateful day.

As I approached the hose tower, I focused intently on regulating my breathing. My heart rate was elevated from all the stairs I had climbed and was about to elevate even higher with this next task. I was mindful that I needed to get my breathing under control. I walked into the hose tower and partnered myself with a dummy. I squatted down and steadied myself as I firmly wrapped my arms around its chest. With force I rose from the squat and hoisted the dummy up to my chest. I drug it through the truck bay as instructed and then out the bay door and onto the ramp. I was about halfway down the ramp when the captain came sauntering up alongside me.

"All you have to do is say, "I quit," Lynnette, and this will all stop," he said ever so casually. "It's as easy as that."

I took a couple more steps and then halted my stride and carefully lowered the dummy to the ground. I wasn't quitting; I was recalibrating. I deliberately turned my head slowly to meet his gaze head-on. I could sense his anticipation for my next move hanging in the air.

"Are you done?" he quietly asked as his eyes bore into mine.

I watched as a smirk tugged at the corners of his mouth. There it was again, a smirk so evil that it sent shivers down my spine. In that moment I felt a surge of defiance rise from within me, and it was the fuel I needed to persevere. Without uttering a word, I turned my head away from him, drew in a slow breath, squatted down with purpose, and forcefully picked the dummy back up. There was no room for surrender and no option but to press on. I would drag this fucking dummy to the ends of the earth today if I had to, just to prove a point.

I couldn't be the only one who saw through his façade. His actions, his words, and his very presence grated against my conscience and left me feeling deeply unsettled. What troubled me most was the collective silence around his behavior. It was as though everyone had agreed to turn a blind eye and pretend it wasn't happening. Not a single person spoke up or took a stand against him. I understood the hierarchical structure of the fire service, where rank commanded respect, but his behavior went far beyond that. It gnawed at me until I came to an unsettling truth. They weren't simply showing respect; they were cowering in fear. It wasn't admiration that kept them silent; it was the oppressive weight of intimidation. In that moment, I realized I wasn't alone in the pervasive atmosphere of fear.

I believe my decision to press on backfired his plan, and the drills stopped after that. Even though the drills ceased, the hostile atmosphere persisted right along with the relentless verbal assaults that were aimed squarely at my presence. He gave me constant reminders that I was on a six-month probation and my fate hung precariously in the balance. He took every opportunity to reinforce the notion that I didn't belong, that I was ill-suited for the role, and that my time within the department was destined for a premature end. I couldn't help but speculate on his motives. Was the desire for my failure merely wishful thinking on his part? Or was he actively scheming behind the scenes and plotting my downfall?

Some days proved to be a difficult battle—not just physically, but mentally and emotionally as well. Through the constant array of challenges and the never-ending hostility, I kept reminding myself that I just had to make the six months. There was that light at the end of the tunnel, and I needed to remain focused. No matter what trials were thrown at me, as long as I fixated on the goal, it would pay off. I convinced myself that once the six-month milestone was surpassed, a new chapter would unfold for me, and things would be different. There would be newfound respect, acceptance, and perhaps even camaraderie. I needed that glimmer of optimism to get me through the darkness.

CHAPTER 10

Oops! I Did It Again

I was well past the midpoint of my probationary period when I reluctantly decided it was probably high time to fulfill my hiring condition of completing the CPAT. *Again.* Having to undergo the ordeal a second time was honestly such a pain in the ass, and I was irritated to no end.

I had completed my consecutive days of training and transitioned to a shift rotation that provided me with greater flexibility to go. My new work schedule followed a four on four off rotation that alternated between two days and two nights, followed by four days off. Once again, at my own expense, I arranged and paid to take the CPAT in Calgary. I kept my plans confidential from the fire department and only told those in my immediate family. It wasn't anyone's business but mine. I felt safer being shielded from external pressures, distractions, and potential discouragement.

This time around, I found myself devoid of any self-doubt or nerves. I felt confident because I was anchored by the knowledge that I was fully capable. My prior experience had affirmed my abilities, both to myself and to them, and it honestly felt ridiculous that I was having to repeat the process.

I followed pretty much the same travel arrangements as I had done the time before. When I arrived at the test facility, I was met by the familiar face of the evaluator from my previous run. His recognition of me was evident and he couldn't help but express his surprise at my return. He was curious about my reappearance, so we chatted briefly about my reasons for coming back to undergo the test once more. I explained the situation and highlighted how my hiring condition mandated my completion of the CPAT for a second time. He shook his head in disbelief, followed by powerful words of encouragement to remind me that I was going to kick ass on it just like I had the time before.

I didn't need any extra prep to psych myself up beforehand as I did before. I entered the testing floor focused and determined to tackle the test with precision and purpose. Being familiar with the course allowed me to navigate it swiftly and optimize my speed anywhere I could to shave off valuable seconds. I completed each event efficiently and finished the test with a surge of strength that came from deep within. There were no tears this time, only a profound sense of pride and ownership that I had earned through sheer effort and determination. When the evaluator revealed the stopwatch, a huge smile spread across my face. I had beat my previous time by a remarkable twenty seconds. The rush of triumph was fucking exhilarating!

After returning home, I resumed my life and work routine like nothing had happened. One day at work I confidently confided in my captain that I had successfully accomplished my CPAT during my days off. He was genuinely happy for me and mirrored my own sentiments toward certain individuals who had doubted me. I think he was more excited than I was about getting to shove it in their faces. I had decided that I didn't want to downplay my achievement by just presenting them with the certificate like it was nothing, because it was something. I recognized its significance, even if they didn't. It wasn't just a piece of paper; it represented my perseverance and triumph over adversity. After having been subjected to the test not once, but twice, while others had been spared, I felt entitled to revel in my success. My probationary period was coming to a close, and I was well aware that speculation was swirling around my ability to complete the test, so I opted to leave them in suspense. I safely stashed the certificate away until I felt it was the perfect moment to unveil it.

The month of May rolled in, signaling the final union meeting before the summer hiatus and meetings being set to resume in September. I was allowed to attend these meetings, but I wasn't allowed to speak on things or vote until I became a sworn member. I couldn't be sworn in until my probation was complete, which loomed only mere days away.

I arrived at the meeting and found an empty chair near the door. I sat quietly and observed the proceedings with a keen ear and absorbed every detail. As the meeting was nearing the end, my captain seized the moment and inquired about the possibility of my induction into the union that night, considering the distant horizon of September. The executive smugly countered that I had not yet completed the CPAT so I could not be inducted. One of the men addressed me directly and asked if I was planning to go and do it, knowing full well that I was pretty much out of time.

"I already did," I responded nonchalantly as I casually retrieved the certificate from my pocket and opened it for display.

The room went silent. One of the men rose from his seat and walked over to take the document from my hand. He stood in place and studied it carefully.

"When did you do this?" he asked.

"A few weeks ago," I casually replied.

With scrutiny he poured back over the document in search of the date. I watched as his eyes met his answer. He turned with the certificate and passed it off to another executive member, who received it with visible irritation.

The once-muted atmosphere had now erupted into whispers and murmurs as a wide range of emotions played out on the faces before me. As I scanned the room, I felt a sense of satisfaction well up inside me at the sight of their disarray. Mid scan, my eyes met my captain's, and he gave me a wink and a smile of approval. Within minutes the executive started to speak, and the air was thick with excuses as they scrambled to rationalize their side. They claimed that because they were caught off guard, they were then ill-prepared to proceed with the ability to swear me in. Their feeble justifications fell short in my eyes. I had witnessed the seamless induction of another member, so I knew firsthand how straightforward the process was. All it entailed was my presence standing before them as they read a simple script, and I answered. That was it. But their composure had clearly shattered in the face of my unexpected triumph. The fact that I had completed the test, unbeknownst to them, seemed to throw them off their game and rendered them incapable of fulfilling what should have been a routine task.

It didn't take long for them to flip the script and shift the blame onto me. They conveniently deflected responsibility for their own lack of preparation. Suddenly, I found myself on the receiving end of their accusations; it was my fault that they were caught off guard, and my fault because they hadn't been informed in advance. They seemed very distressed over my supposed betrayal and demanded an explanation as to why I had kept my CPAT success a secret from them. My response was as straightforward as it was unapologetic. It was none of their fucking business! Contrary to their beliefs, they were not entitled to know until now.

As a result, my wait to be sworn into the union stretched out for an additional four months until the September meeting. I harbored some concerns that my status of being a non-sworn member left me in a vulnerable position, but I was assured that wasn't the case. With probation behind me, I officially held a place within the fire department, so I was supposedly shielded by the union's umbrella of protection. However, my past encounters had left me somewhat skeptical about whether their idea of safeguarding and mine were the same thing. All I could do at this point was hope that my need for their protection would remain a distant hypothetical rather than a grim reality.

CHAPTER 11

You Never Forget Your First

I was comfortably settling into my shift and gradually bonding with my new crew mates. Each day brought new experiences and challenges. From dispatching a variety of emergencies, to responding to multiple fire calls, and—unfortunately—attending my first fatality.

I was working a night shift, and the early morning air was filled with the wails of sirens from both police and ambulances. We stood by in anticipation, waiting for our call, but it didn't come. We were all a little disappointed; responding to calls of duty and assisting in emergencies made us feel useful. But instead, we continued with our usual morning routine, and I went on to take care of some station duties.

A significant length of time later, a call came into dispatch for a single-vehicle rollover with unknown entrapment. The uncertainty meant we could attend, and I felt a rush of excitement because I was on the truck this time.

We quickly geared up and three of us loaded into the rescue truck, which was our designated apparatus for motor vehicle incidents. I was in the driver's seat, carefully navigating code 3 through town and out onto the highway. Approximately ten minutes later we came up on the scene. As we approached, dispatch updated us that entrapment was confirmed. This immediately heightened our urgency and frustration as we knew that time was critical, and we had been dispatched very late to the call.

As we arrived, I noticed a retired member of our department and an ambulance crew already on scene. One vehicle was upside down in a ditch and surrounded by multiple people. We parked strategically to block traffic and rushed to assess the vehicle. The retired member informed us that one patient was pinned under the car, alert and responsive. Our captain directed us to quickly assemble the necessary extrication tools while he completed a thorough scene assessment.

Once the tools were ready and our captain returned, we gathered as a team and quickly devised a plan. We strategically placed cribbing to secure the vehicle and ensure everyone's safety. Due to the unique placement of the patient, we had chosen to use airbags to lift the vehicle off her. Each of us assumed our position, and before we began I introduced myself to the patient and asked her name. Throughout the operation I verbally updated her on each step. I didn't have a visual on her, so I was ensuring that she was still responding, but also aware of what was happening.

We soon freed enough space to extricate her to a safe space where we could administer medical attention. However, as soon as we moved her, she went into cardiac arrest. This was my first time performing CPR on a human being and it was vastly different from practicing on a mannequin. My colleague and I took turns performing chest compressions and managing her airway while the paramedics worked swiftly on other lifesaving interventions.

We worked tirelessly, but despite our best efforts, she succumbed to her injuries. I watched as my colleague gently covered her exposed body to show her the dignity she deserved. We all paused in a silent, unspoken moment of respect. I had never been on the scene of a fatality before and had only ever dispatched for one, so I was unsure of what to do. I decided to follow the lead of my colleague and my captain's directions.

We cleaned up our equipment and returned it to the truck. I found myself glancing repeatedly at the covered body lying motionless in the grass. I was feeling a complex mix of emotions but was uncertain how to process them. Until that moment, I had been entirely focused on the task at hand and relied on my training and captain to guide me through the call. There hadn't been time to come to terms with what was happening until now, but I didn't even want to do that until we were clear of the scene.

We remained there for quite some time, awaiting the coroner. My captain spoke with me privately several times to check on my well-being and answer my numerous questions. It was all very new to me, so he helped me understand the procedures and protocols that were being followed.

Once we were given permission to clear, we returned to the firehall. During the drive back our captain was very gracious in giving each of us time to speak on what we had experienced. Upon our return, my captain spoke with me once more before I left for home. I was being honest when I assured him that I felt okay. I arrived home, had breakfast, and went to bed, able to sleep as I normally did. I had been warned that the experience might haunt me, but it didn't. My lack of emotional turmoil was what troubled me the most. Why was I not feeling anything? I was almost afraid it would jump out at me later, like a scene from a suspenseful horror movie. I felt myself anticipating the emotional fallout, but it never came.

To address my concerns, I made an appointment with my counselor. It was an enlightening session where I learned that it was normal not to feel emotionally impacted every time I encountered a tragedy. I realized that I had relied heavily on my training to navigate the call and had subconsciously disconnected myself emotionally. I had been told two pieces of advice in the very beginning of my career. Don't look in the patient's eyes, if possible, as they are the window to the soul. And always remember that I wasn't there and didn't cause the accident. Unbeknownst to me, that advice had enabled me to maintain a professional focus.

As I understood this, I was able to give myself grace for not feeling distressed post-call. I had used a personal safety measure on scene, and now a healthy coping mechanism with my counselling appointment. I knew in that moment that I would be okay doing this job.

I had been told that you never forget your first and I can attest to that statement. I would never forget the details of that fateful day.

Nor would I ever forget the details of my first child fatality that followed shortly thereafter. It shook me to my core in a way I hadn't anticipated. When we arrived at the scene of the motor vehicle incident, we were all taken aback by our initial assessment, as there had been no prior warning of a child being involved. We quickly discovered that both a mother and her young son were deceased, and no medical interventions were necessary.

The accident occurred on a busy highway, so we immediately began performing traffic control until the coroner arrived. After some time, we received an update that the coroner was going to be delayed and that we would be released from the scene for now. We were instructed to return when the coroner arrived. In the meantime, the highway was shut down to allow the police to complete their investigation and reenactment of the incident.

It was a haunting feeling, knowing that I had to go back to the scene. Initially responding, seeing everything, getting to work, and then leaving was one thing. But having to return, knowing full well what I was coming back to, and seeing it all over again was a completely different experience.

A few hours later we were called back to the scene. When we arrived, we were met by the coroner, who gave us instructions on what he needed us to do. While he was completing his examinations, we donned our PPE and set up our tools. Shortly thereafter, I was hands-on to strategically extricate both the mother and the boy from the wreckage. Carefully placing his small body into a body bag was unlike anything I had ever experienced, and something I would never forget. The weight of the tragedy was palpable, and the images of that day would stay with me forever. The somber atmosphere, the stillness of the scene, and the gravity of the loss etched themselves into my memory. The innocence of a child being taken so abruptly and unfairly challenged my sense of justice and left a lasting impact.

Unfortunately, my career was soon marked by an overwhelming number of traumatic scenes and encounters with deceased individuals. The sheer volume of fatalities I attended over the years was staggering, far beyond what I had anticipated. Each incident etched a new scar on my soul. Yet no matter how many times I faced the grim reality of death I remained committed to my role, driven by a sense of duty and the desire to help others in their most critical moments.

CHAPTER 12

"Women Belong At Home"

There were some sobering realities of the job, but I was fully immersed in my new career and loving it. I was expanding my knowledge base continuously and approaching each day with an open mind and a willingness to learn. I didn't have a mechanical background of any kind, and I was driving and operating all the fire apparatus. That in and of itself was a massive undertaking. I was learning the ins and outs of what to do on a fire scene and at the site of motor vehicle incidents. I took every opportunity to absorb information and actively participate in the steep learning curve that came with my role.

The firehall was old and posed a unique challenge for a female firefighter like me. Unlike the facilities back in Texas, there were no separate amenities tailored to accommodate my needs; no separate washroom, shower, or locker room for getting changed. It required some creative adjustments on my part. I would arrive at work already clad in my uniform to eliminate the need for a dedicated changing area. If I had plans post-shift, I would have to change into my street clothes in the bathroom. Not ideal but it sufficed. I never voiced any grievances or aired my concerns to anyone because it was pointless when they were logistical hurdles imposed by the outdated infrastructure. If I needed to go into the locker room, I always enlisted one of the guys to check first to respect everyone's privacy and make sure no one was changing. Even a routine trip to the washroom and an open door meant a precautionary knock and vocal announcement to ensure it was empty. I didn't want any surprises! It was a constant dance of vigilance to avoid intruding on anyone's personal space. A dance some of the guys blatantly refused to learn, while others just naturally fell into step. The reality was clear: the building wasn't designed with a female in mind, and renovations were simply out of the question. I didn't expect any preferential treatment, and I didn't want to make things awkward or disrupt the harmony of the team. So I made do with what I had.

During night shifts, once our tasks were completed and the station fell into a temporary lull between calls, we were granted the luxury of rest. However, the sleeping arrangements left much to be desired with one cramped room that housed three twin beds, and the captain in solitary quarters in the room next door. One particular night there were only three of us on duty, as the captain had the night off. The most senior member assumed command as the acting captain and had the privilege of the captain's room as his own.

However, his authority took a baffling turn when he declared that it wasn't appropriate for a woman to share a room with a man, just the two of them. Without consulting me or raising the issue directly, he took it upon himself to declare that the other firefighter was not allowed to stay in the room with me. I was completely unaware of the conversation that had transpired, so I didn't put much thought into the other firefighter's actions when he grabbed his things and slept on the couch. After all, it wasn't uncommon for some of the guys to seek alternative sleeping arrangements from time to time. However, the next morning revealed an awkward tension in the air, short answers, and a prickly attitude directed at me. I was confused by the sudden change, so I asked my colleague numerous times what was going on, and the only answer I received insinuated that I should already know. That didn't sit well with me, so I continued probing for answers, only to find out that it was suggested that I was somehow responsible for the discomfort and perceived impropriety of us sharing a room. What? That couldn't have been further from the truth! I quickly clarified my stance and emphasized that I had absolutely no reservations about sharing sleeping quarters with anyone, and any perceived issue lay solely on the acting captain's opinion and judgement. I had more than enough confidence in my integrity and character to know for certain that I would never partake in or initiate any inappropriate behavior. I had a very candid conversation with the other firefighter and calmly claimed my innocence with the unnecessary turmoil that had unfolded. I was grateful we were able to hash out our grievances and reach a mutual understanding of clarity. It was a relief that he listened and ultimately chose to believe me. It pained me that a simple misunderstanding had spiraled into unnecessary drama and strained the relations between us. I was angry because I had worked hard to build trust and acceptance, and that acting captain had done a lot of damage in a short period of time. Now I had to be the one to put back together what he had undone.

We came back on shift the next night, and things for me felt tense and awkward. I kept myself busy out in the truck bays with pump familiarization and cleaning. I had pulled the rescue truck outside and was cleaning equipment when the acting captain approached me. He gave me a quick apology but followed it with an explanation that he held firm to the belief that the fire department wasn't a suitable place for a woman. He asserted that he stood by the notion that a man and woman shouldn't be in a bedroom alone together. I didn't say anything; I simply studied him while he spoke.

"A woman belongs at home, and you being here is only an invitation for trouble," he explained.

He spoke his truth with conviction, and he stood strong in his perspective. He followed up by asking me what kind of point I was trying to prove by being there. I contemplated even responding because it felt like a loaded question, but I opted for the same level of honesty he had just offered me.

"I don't have a point to prove. I want to contribute to the team and serve my community," I stated. "Why is that so hard to understand?"

He didn't answer me.

I had no intention of overshadowing or weakening anyone. Nor did I seek to cause trouble or disrupt any relationships. I had no romantic interest in any of my male colleagues! My intentions were purely selfish in the pursuit of knowledge and growth. That appeared to be a difficult concept for others to grasp but it was honestly all I wanted! There was a wealth of collective experience within the department, and I simply wanted to absorb as much wisdom from them as possible so I could become an exemplary firefighter.

I wasn't heard. I gave my best efforts to express my perspective, but it seemed that our exchange only led to a stalemate. We had to agree to disagree and leave it at that. Our inability to bridge the gap left me feeling wounded. His misconceptions about me really stung. I had lost respect for him. His rigid beliefs were his and he owned them. I had accepted his apology even though it was accompanied by a "but" and the whole issue was left unresolved.

Due to the severity of the situation, it was brought to the chief's attention—not by me—and it was dealt with at that level. A week later I was called into the chief's office to provide my perspective, and I recounted the events as they had transpired. I was told that the acting captain had been given a warning because his behavior bordered on discriminatory conduct and there could be disciplinary action. I was asked if I would like to pursue any sort of formal action, and I opted against it. I didn't want to escalate the conflict, and I sure as hell didn't need any further fallout. All I wanted was a professional workplace where this sort of nonsense didn't arise again.

In the end, the incident was swept under the rug, with everyone moving on like it never happened. Yet for me, the memory lingered, and I couldn't move past it. So, I took it upon myself to ensure extra comfort for everyone else within the team. Whenever circumstances arose where only two of us would be occupying a room, I made a point to seek reassurance from them that they felt comfortable with the situation. I would've slept elsewhere if they didn't.

Throughout all my years in the firehall, I never had another issue like that from anyone else. Whether he was the only one who believed it strongly enough to voice it, or whether he was a lone soldier in his way of thinking, I'll never know. Working alongside the guys demanded a level of cooperation and camaraderie, and navigating delicate situations wasn't easy, but it always ended with compromise. It often required me to let grievances slide and divert my attention elsewhere for the sake of preserving the collective peace.

But it was never my peace I was keeping.

CHAPTER 13

I Promise I Won't Be *That* Girl

"We're not coming to save you. You're on your own." Those words had etched themselves into the very core of my being and were a constant haunting reminder of betrayal. They were more than just words to me; they were a dagger to my soul, and a terrifying realization that in the most critical moments, I could be left to die without the support of my colleagues. Before that moment of threat, I had never feared death. Now, fear consumed me.

How could I possibly thrive in my profession with that in the shadows of my mind? This wasn't just any profession; it was one where every decision held the weight of life and death! The answer was simple: I couldn't. How could I muster the courage to excel, to push my limits, and to reach my full potential when I was crippled by fear? Again, I couldn't.

With every call I responded to, its presence loomed in the shadows. It was like a perpetual caution sign hanging over me, urging me to proceed with the utmost care. As a result, I engaged in a constant stream of self-talk, reminding me to stay vigilant.

"Okay, watch what you're doing. Don't make any stupid moves. Don't mess things up. Breathe. Stay focused. You can do this!"

These pep talks became my lifeline as I worked each task. My mind was consumed with the fear of making a wrong move. I prayed with every fiber of my being that I wouldn't get into any kind of trouble or harmful situation because I was terrified by the possibly that his warnings might hold truth. The toll was immense, and it fucked with me mentally, emotionally, and physically.

I failed to grasp it at the time but owning that captains' actions had bred a host of limiting beliefs within me. I was hesitant to take risks and showcase my abilities, which held me back from discovering my full potential. This self-imposed restraint deprived not only myself but also my department, my colleagues, and my community of the opportunity to witness the extent of my capabilities and was ultimately a huge disservice to us all.

Silently, I was battling an internal conflict that I kept hidden from everyone. The conversation from that day remained locked within me and was a secret that I dared not to share. Why? Because I believed that speaking out would have jeopardized my position and prevented me from making it through my probation. The man behind that conversation had already gone to great lengths in attempting to sabotage my initial hiring, so I truly feared that he possessed the power to curtail my career before it even got started. As a result, I remained silent and bore the weight of my apprehensions alone.

Prior to my hiring, there had been unsettling news reports circulating from a few fire departments that had hired female firefighters and were embroiled in lawsuits due to discrimination, harassment, and bullying. The stories of the treatment the women endured while on the job were horrific, and the trauma they experienced for speaking out was disturbing. I was devastated to learn one woman ended her life because of it. It was all unacceptable! Yet within my own department, the echoes of misogyny were loud. There were numerous discussions and the conversations were fierce. Some of the men voiced sentiments like, "That's what happens when you hire a female. Trouble follows." They were very concerned that my presence would only invite trouble. I reassured them, and solemnly swore that I would never disrupt the harmony of the department. There were many of them, and only one of me, and here I was making it my mission to ensure that they were comfortable and confident that I wasn't going to turn on them and cause them any trouble.

I stuck to my promise because I never wanted to be "that girl." The girl who caused trouble, who made waves, and who tarnished the reputation of others. From the beginning I reassured myself that things weren't as dire as they appeared, and I excused and dismissed the mistreatment and unacceptable behaviors I encountered. I told myself that I possessed the resilience to endure whatever came my way, and then somewhere along the way I convinced myself that if I couldn't handle what was happening, then I was weak. I had been exposed to domineering and abusive men from a young age, which had desensitized me to such treatment, so this was a familiar, albeit unwelcome, reality. I had survived men like them—and worse—through various stages my whole life. My strategy? I refused to engage or react to starve their toxicity of the attention it craved, hoping they would eventually tire and stop.

Rather than vocalizing my objections, I chose to absorb everything they hurled my way. I wore an outward facade of indifference and was determined not to give them the satisfaction of seeing me affected by their misogynistic attitudes and self-centered antics. I was very aware of my outnumbered position, so I opted for the path of least resistance where I would just pretend and play along nicely. It was nothing more than a draining and emotionally taxing survival strategy.

I worked hard to exceed their expectations and often went the extra mile just to ensure they wouldn't have any grounds for criticism against me. They could never accuse me of being defiant, a bitch, or impolite. I was a good girl. I extended kindness to them even when they were ignorant fucks to me. I listened even when they yelled. I didn't talk back even when I knew they were wrong. And I did my job even when they made it extra.

I spent well over a decade trying to prove myself worthy. I was under constant scrutiny, with watchful eyes eagerly anticipating any misstep they could use against me. It was an endless, exhausting pursuit to validate myself that created so much self-doubt that it broke my confidence.

Deep down I knew that firefighting was my true calling. I possessed the skills and the passion to excel in the role, if given the opportunity. Yes, there were instances where I was able to showcase my abilities and shine brightly, but not to the degree that I should've been able to throughout my career.

CHAPTER 14

My Secret Existence

On more than one occasion, I was contacted by local and provincial media, who were intrigued by the significance of my role as the first female firefighter in Dawson Creek. They were requesting an interview with me so they could run a story. I was uncertain of the department's protocols regarding media interviews, so I sought the guidance of my captain, who enthusiastically supported the idea and encouraged me to consult with management and the union. While management offered no objections, the response from the union and a few others was another story. I was unexpectedly confronted by two of my union executive members one afternoon out in the truck bay.

"What is this we're hearing about you wanting to talk to the media?" Their words and tone were laced with intimidation. "If you were smart, you wouldn't do that."

Vastly overstepping their authority, I was threatened with disciplinary action and possible termination if I was ever caught speaking to them. They made it very clear that I would not receive support from the union or my brothers if I defied their warning. Shockingly, the narrative had been twisted to portray me as seeking personal attention at the department's expense, and they weren't going to stand for it.

I was extremely confused and filled with inner turmoil, but I obediently complied with their directive. Whenever I was contacted by the media, I followed the same script, claiming there was no story to tell and that I was declining to provide any further comments. Deep down I grappled with regret and sadness over a missed opportunity. I had encountered many news headlines where departments were announcing the hiring of their first female firefighter and read countless articles where they proudly celebrated her and commended her on blazing a trail. They were excited about the addition of a female and welcomed her with open arms. I couldn't help but wonder what that kind of support and inclusion would feel like.

It deeply saddened me that they didn't want the public to know about my presence or accomplishments. I wasn't seeking attention at the department's expense. I genuinely believed that sharing my story would have cast a positive light on both the department and our small town. As I reflected on the situation, it became apparent that their resistance stemmed from an inability to look beyond their egos and recognize the potential benefits for everyone. Publicly acknowledging my achievements could have boosted the department's image and garnered respect for them as progressive leaders. But doing so would have required them to give me some recognition, and that was a concession they were unwilling to make.

One day while working at the firehall, my phone rang from an unknown number. Normally, I wouldn't answer such calls, but for some reason I did.

"Hello," I cautiously greeted.

"Hello, I was wondering if I could have a moment of your time." He immediately began complimenting me and congratulating me on becoming a firefighter.

I was grateful for his kind words, so I thanked him and then asked who I was speaking to. He introduced himself by providing both his name and then his title. He was a reporter from a media station that wasn't local. I instantly froze as his words began to blur together.

"I'm curious if you have experienced any discrimination or harassment as the only female firefighter at the station?" he asked.

Completely caught off guard, I panicked and hung up the phone. I nervously looked over my shoulder in fear that someone may have heard what was asked, then gave a sigh of relief when I discovered I was alone in the truck bay. I stood there for a moment, staring off into the distance, my mind racing with questions. Why had he asked me that? Was it assumed that I would face discrimination and harassment as the only female firefighter? Had he been tipped off about something specific and was now trying to verify it? Or was he just curious if my experience might mirror those of women in other departments? I didn't know the answers, but his question had seemed odd. Seeds of curiosity were now planted in my mind.

It didn't go away, and the more I thought about the conversation, the more it sparked a different perspective within me. I began to wonder if the department's insistence on keeping me away from the media had a more self-serving motive. The fact that they were so adamant about keeping me hidden and silent made me think that they were trying to protect themselves and prevent any uncomfortable truths from being exposed.

CHAPTER 15

That's What Happens When You Hire A Female

After my divorce, I went through a series of failed relationships, always finding myself drawn to the wrong men—those who were either emotionally unavailable or simply not right for me. Each new relationship felt like an uphill battle and the idea of starting over became exhausting. I eventually reached a point where I swore off dating altogether and actually felt content with being single. However, a persistent friend of mine wouldn't take no for an answer and was determined to set me up with her neighbor, a man she insisted was perfect for me. Despite my reluctance, she kept pushing, and after I canceled our first scheduled date—and he canceled the second—I finally agreed to the third just to get her off my back. She even convinced me by joking that, at the very least, I'd get a free meal out of it. I met him at a local restaurant, and to my surprise, we clicked right away. The conversation was easy, and he turned out to be kind, funny, and genuinely interested in getting to know me. What started as a reluctant blind date turned into a real connection and we continued dating from that day forward.

I had been working full-time at the fire department for roughly a year and a half when I made the decision to close my hair salon. Juggling two full-time jobs left me completely drained, with little to no time for a personal life, let alone a serious relationship. It was a bittersweet choice—my salon had been a passion project, but firefighting had become my calling. In the end, something had to give, and I chose to open space in my life for something more meaningful.

We had been engaged for just over a year, and my fiancé and I were putting the final touches on our wedding plans. We were getting married on the picturesque beach on Grand Cayman Island and it was a dream destination. The departure date was nearing, and we were immersed in the excitement of carefully selecting every detail to make our wedding day perfect. I couldn't wait! The azure waters, the soft white sand, and the gentle island breeze was going to be the perfect backdrop for our vows. Then, just before we left, we received a surprise that would make our special day even more unforgettable. A special guest would be joining us at our wedding; we were expecting a baby! The news was both shocking and thrilling and added a special layer of joy to our already momentous occasion.

Deep down, I was panicking, but I managed to keep my focus on the wedding and enjoy the day. Our wedding turned out to be everything we had dreamed of. It was beautiful and intimate. The ceremony was simple and elegant, with us barefoot on a private section of beach just like we had envisioned. The soft sand beneath our feet and the gentle rhythm of the waves created a serene and magical atmosphere. My stepson joined us for the trip, which added a special touch to the celebration. We were also fortunate to invite a couple of close friends who lived on the island and together with my stepson made up our small but meaningful wedding party.

The ceremony itself was perfect. We exchanged vows under the clear blue sky with the ocean as our backdrop and the breeze gently rustling through the palm trees. There were no elaborate decorations or grand gestures, just the natural beauty of the island and the genuine love we shared. It was exactly what we had envisioned.

After the wedding we indulged in a mini honeymoon on the island and savored every moment of our newlywed bliss. We explored the local sights, enjoyed the amazing food, and spent time at the pool and along the gorgeous beach. Each day was filled with celebration, not only for our marriage but also the exciting news of our growing family. Returning home, we were filled with joy and anticipation for the future. We had beautiful memories of our day on Grand Cayman Island that would forever be cherished and marked the beginning of a new chapter in our lives. A chapter that promised adventure, love, and the start of our family journey.

Once I was back at home, reality hit me hard. The euphoria of the wedding and the honeymoon began to fade and was replaced by the sobering realization of what lay ahead. My career as a firefighter wasn't safe at the best of times, let alone while pregnant. The thought of continuing in such a physically demanding and hazardous role while carrying a child was overwhelming. I couldn't grasp how I was going to manage it, or even what my next steps should be. Panic had fully set in as I thought about the risks involved in my job. The heavy lifting, the exposure to toxic smoke and chemicals, and the unpredictable nature of emergency calls. My mind raced with questions and fears. How could I protect my baby while fulfilling my duties? Was there a way to balance both my career and my impending motherhood? How long would I be able to work with a growing belly? I was making myself more anxious and fearful with every unanswered question. I knew that I couldn't navigate this foreign territory alone. The first thing I needed to do was inform the chief. I had to let him know about my pregnancy so he could hopefully provide me with some guidance and direction on what would happen next. It was scary because I knew this was uncharted territory for both me and the department, so I only hoped that they would have policies in place to support me.

I was scheduled to be back on shift, so I got to work and did my best to start the day as usual. But the weight of my news made it impossible to maintain my normal routine for very long. As soon as I could, I approached the chief's office. My whole body was shaking, and I was teetering on the verge of tears. Why was I so nervous? Here I was, a grown woman, yet I felt like a teenager who was about to deliver some bad news to her parents. As I approached his office, he looked up from his desk and smiled. I had summoned all my courage, yet when I spoke my voice was shaky.

"Are you available to chat?" I asked.

He nodded and motioned for me to come in. I wanted to step forward, but my legs felt too wobbly to carry me any farther, so I stood by the door and used the frame to steady myself.

"How was the wedding?" he asked. "Congratulations."

I shared a few details and thanked him for his kind words. Then, with my heart pounding, I told him that I also had some other news. He looked up at me questioningly. And as soon as our eyes met, the tears I had been holding back started to fall.

"I'm pregnant!" I blurted out.

His face lit up with genuine joy.

"Congratulations! That's great news," he said. "Isn't it?"

I think it was difficult for him to tell because the tears were streaming down my face. It was good news, but it was also terrifying. I loved my career and had no idea what this would mean for me and firefighting. We talked briefly about my concerns, and the chief offered nothing but reassurance. He explained that he needed to inform the union and they would sort some things out. He promised we would figure out the details together and encouraged me not to worry. I gave him permission to share the news with them, wiped the tears from my face, and prepared myself for the next step: telling the rest of my crew. I wanted them to hear it from me directly. I was still an emotional wreck, so I went to the washroom to try to pull myself together. I found my captain and the rest of my crew out in the bay, and as soon as they saw me, they looked extremely concerned. I told them I needed to talk, and they gathered quickly as they sensed the gravity of what I was about to share. It took me a minute, but I finally managed to get the words out and told them straight up that I was pregnant. Their response was immediate and overwhelmingly positive. Smiles spread across their faces, and they enveloped me in hugs and offered huge congratulations. Their happiness for me was genuine and it helped ease my anxiety.

Word spread like wildfire, of course. This was big news. There was obviously no way of keeping it a secret until I was in the safe zone of twelve weeks. Almost immediately, I received an outpouring of heartfelt congratulations. Many of my colleagues were genuinely happy for me and expressed their support and excitement for this new chapter in my life. However, not everyone was so kind. As expected, a few chauvinistic and inconsiderate comments surfaced.

"This is what happens when you hire a female!"

My brain was fired up. Because I was a woman, my pregnancy was an inconvenience they should have anticipated.

I was quietly doing my duties when I was cornered by one of the men.

"Has the chief decided on a plan for you yet, because I can't work with you being like *that*," he said, making a dismissive gesture toward my stomach.

I looked to where he was pointing and laid a hand across my belly, quietly shaking my head from side to side. I wasn't even showing yet.

The comment that stung the most came from a particularly outspoken captain who approached me with a sneer. "No one wanted to work with you before, and now you've made things way worse for yourself," he said. "Everyone will be keeping their distance from you because they sure as hell aren't going to be taking the blame for your baby getting hurt." He shook his head. "What the fuck were you thinking?"

Then he turned and walked away. His words cut deep. Just as he had intended. The implication that my pregnancy made me a liability was infuriating and disheartening.

I had no answers for any of the questions they fired at me. As they voiced their opinions and concerns for themselves at various times, all I could do was listen. Their words surrounded me like a storm and there was a constant barrage of chatter from every direction. Conversations took place in front of me, behind me, to me, and about me. Once again, I was the talk of the firehall. Or maybe I had never stopped being the subject of their discussions. Either way, I was undeniably in the spotlight. *Again.*

One afternoon, the situation took a particularly uncomfortable turn. I was called into the chief's office.

"The union wants proof of your pregnancy," he stated. "Can you get a letter from your doctor?"

I was dumbfounded. But agreed.

I called my doctor's office and explained the situation to the nurse, outlining the bizarre request I had received. She immediately informed me I was under no legal obligation to provide proof of my pregnancy.

"Shame on them for even asking," she added, her voice tinged with disapproval.

I thanked her for her insight and hung up the phone. But despite her reassurance, I felt a mix of emotions stirring inside me. Part of me wanted to just give them the proof, if only to settle the issue and put their doubts to rest. Yet a deeper, more outraged part of me resented that they were questioning my integrity, once again forcing me to go above and beyond what was right—just to put their minds at ease. The implication that I needed to prove something so personal felt like a violation—an insult.

I went back to the chief and relayed what the nurse had told me. He listened carefully, nodding in understanding. He would forward the information to the union executives and seemed confident this would resolve the issue once and for all. I left his office hoping it was a closed case.

As I made my way back to the truck bay, one of my colleagues noticed the frustration on my face.

"Hey, are you okay?" he asked, his tone filled with concern.

"Not really," I replied, not holding back. "The union wanted proof of my pregnancy, but legally I don't have to provide it."

He paused for a moment before responding and what came next completely blindsided me. "Why wouldn't you just give it to them anyway?"

I stared at him, stunned.

"Are you serious?" I asked, trying to process his words.

"If you're really pregnant then you should have no problem proving it," he said, his tone casual, as if what he was suggesting was perfectly reasonable. "What's the big deal?"

I couldn't believe what I was hearing. Anger was starting to move through me. This was a man I felt I could trust for support, but I was seeing a side of him I never imagined existed.

"This conversation is over," I said, my voice hard and final.

Without waiting for a response, I turned and walked away, my emotions simmering just below the surface.

In the end, the chief had been right—the case was closed and the matter of proving my pregnancy was never brought up again. But I often wondered how far the union executives had gone in their efforts before finally realizing their demand was not only intrusive but also unlawful.

It had always been drilled into me that everything revolved around "the contract." It was the ultimate authority and ruler of all things. But much to my dismay, there was nothing in it regarding maternity leave. Since there had never been a female firefighter in the department, there was no mention of provisions for one anywhere in the contract. Even though I had been a member of the union for over two years now, they still hadn't changed or updated anything. The entire contract was still written exclusively for men, with no language to incorporate a "sister" in the brotherhood. The issue of it needing to be changed had come up in conversations, but it was always quickly dismissed and confirmed that nothing would be done until the next contract negotiation. Meanwhile, I was given lip service that I had nothing to worry about and was covered under the contract, even with the glaring omissions.

Now here I was, pregnant and feeling extremely vulnerable and insecure because there was nothing in writing to cover me. The most pressing question I had was whether I would have a job to return to after my maternity leave. Given our history, I always felt the need to cover all my bases to mitigate any potential threats with these guys. I had zero trust in them to look out for my best interests. The contract included details covering men for the day of birth and paternity leave, but nothing for the mother giving birth and maternity leave.

I followed protocol and brought my questions to one of my union representatives. I listened as he spoke and didn't have a good feeling about the information he was stating. His answers were far too quick and most of them didn't make any sense. I left that meeting feeling more confused than when I had gone in—as if I was on my own. My suspicions were confirmed when I did some digging and discovered that much of what he had told me was inaccurate. He didn't know the answers to any of my questions, yet he sure tried to sound like he did. None of that was helpful and added immensely to my stress.

I was determined to find some clarity, so I had several meetings with my other union executives. I felt exposed and afraid about my future with the department after my baby was born but I still didn't get any solid answers. I realized I needed to take matters into my own hands, so I reached out to another woman I knew who wasn't in the fire service but was the president of her union. She provided me with some incredible support and advised me to speak to my shop steward, who was supposed to help me. I was grateful for her direction and irritated that no one within my own union had suggested that. But I was armed with this new information now, so I reached out to my shop steward and asked for his assistance. Thankfully, he was very receptive and resourceful. He admitted that he didn't know any of the answers, but he was going to find them. It didn't take him long to come back to me with a wealth of information he had dug into from legal rights and labor codes. He discovered that I would, in fact, be secure despite the lack of specific provisions in the contract. I was entitled to maternity leave. I didn't have to pay union dues while I was away. I would hold my seniority, and I had a job to come back to. Having these answers was a huge relief and lifted a tremendous weight off my shoulders. The stress of being a terrified pregnant woman trying to secure her future in a male-dominated field was overwhelming. Knowing that I was finally safe allowed me to relax a little.

The brief moment of relaxation quickly vanished when I learned that two of my union brothers were blatantly betraying "the brotherhood" and actively pressuring the chief to fire me—undermining everything the union was supposed to stand for. Their argument was based on the belief that, due to my pregnancy, I was no longer capable of performing my duties as a firefighter. They felt that I was being given special treatment and therefore campaigning for my employment to be terminated. It was made abundantly clear to both of them, however, that firing me simply for being pregnant was not only against the law but also ethically wrong. They were warned about treading on dangerous ground when they threatened to push the issue higher. It didn't appear to take long however before the matter faded into the background as I had the sense that their misguided attempt to have me removed had hit a dead end.

As my pregnancy progressed, I continued working, though it was agreed that I would no longer be attending the scenes during calls to ensure the safety of myself and others. My growing belly made it difficult to don my gear quickly, and I was unable to perform some of the physical tasks that I used to handle with ease. I felt like I was missing out, and I truly loved being in on the action. But I knew that I could potentially pose a risk, so I had to be content to stay back at the firehall where I took on the role of dispatcher during calls. This position was a safe environment that still allowed me to contribute significantly to our operations without exposing myself or my unborn child to potential dangers. I was determined to keep working as long as possible before the baby's arrival and the dispatching duties allowed me to do just that.

I was six and a half months pregnant, and everything had been progressing smoothly. I was still very active and managing my work duties effectively. One early morning as I was getting ready for work, I walked into the kitchen to prepare my breakfast. As I approached the counter, I suddenly felt something unusual. I looked down and was horrified to see blood dripping onto the floor from beneath my housecoat. I froze for a moment, struggling to comprehend what was happening. When the connection hit me, panic set in instantly. I rushed to the bathroom, where I hoped to get a clearer sense of the situation. Upon investigation, the sight that greeted me was alarming; I was bleeding heavily. I was alone and terrified, and wanted to scream for help, but there was no one else at home. I desperately needed to calm myself so I could try to think through the next steps. I began talking out loud, trying to problem solve what was happening and what I should be doing besides panicking. Terror was surging through my body, and I felt desperate for my unborn child. With trembling hands, I grabbed my phone and called my husband, who was away at work. With each unanswered call, my anxiety grew more intense. He was unreachable, and I had no other way to contact him at his location. I was panicked and desperate. I paced back and forth across the room, trying to decide who I should call next. I opted to call my father because he lived nearby and prayed out loud that he would answer. To my immense relief, he answered immediately, and I broke down in tears. Between sobs I explained the situation and my plan to drive myself to the hospital. He questioned if I was able to drive myself and then assured me he would meet me there as quickly as possible. I hung up the phone and quickly scanned a list of people in my head. I briefly debated calling my mother next, but she lived out of town on a farm and wouldn't be able to get to me quickly, so I decided to call her later. Next, I dialed my captain and woke him from a deep sleep. I hastily explained the emergency and that I wasn't going to be at work because I was going to the hospital. My voice was shaking with fear. I didn't have anyone left to call, so I quickly and carefully got dressed and made my way out of the house and into the car. I drove to the hospital with urgency, treating stop signs as yield signs and exceeding speed limits to get there as fast as possible.

Upon checking in, the hospital staff acted swiftly. They placed me in a wheelchair and rushed me to the maternity ward where a flurry of activity surrounded me as I was hooked up to several monitors. After running some tests, they determined that I was having contractions and was in early labor, which was hard to comprehend because I wasn't feeling any contractions. The printout from the monitors, however, showed a different story. The doctor soon arrived and gave me concerning news. The hospital in my small town was not equipped to handle premature births, so they were in contact with larger medical centers to find a suitable facility for me. I was told that I would need to be flown by air ambulance to a hospital that could provide the necessary care for both me and the baby. The entire day was spent organizing the facility and the transfer; ultimately, Vancouver was chosen as my destination. This was not the news I wanted to hear, as Vancouver was twelve hours away by car, and I would be making this journey alone.

Throughout the day, I kept my family and colleagues updated on the evolving situation. Finally, my husband managed to return my calls. He was working two provinces away near the USA border, where cell service was virtually nonexistent. He had gone to bed after the night shift and was shocked to find an overwhelming number of missed calls and voicemails from me when he woke. He listened intently and absorbed all the details of what had happened and the urgent steps we now needed to take. My husband was in a remote location, five hours away from the nearest city with an airport. He hadn't slept much, but he immediately began making calls and arrangements to leave work and organize his travel to Vancouver, arriving the following day.

I had left the house in such a panic that morning that I didn't have anything with me. Realizing my predicament, I asked a friend to go to my house and pack a bag of essentials for me. I texted her a list of what I thought might be important and then gave her directions on where to find specific things in my house. It was a very challenging task to organize everything under such stress and within such a limited timeframe. I instructed her to gather basics like clothing, toiletries, and a few comfort items that I felt could help me through the hospital stay. I knew it was impossible to cover all my needs in that moment and accepted that I might forget something. My friend did her best to follow my instructions and I was grateful for her help during this crisis. This frantic coordination added another layer of stress to an already overwhelming situation but knowing I would have some of my belongings with me provided a much-needed measure of comfort.

As dinner approached, I finally received confirmation that a plane was coming for me. The reality of the situation hit me hard, and I was gripped by fear. I texted a few colleagues at the firehall to update them and received a couple of unexpected and surprising texts of well-wishes from a few others. My mom was with me at the hospital and offered strong words of encouragement through our teary goodbyes. It broke my heart that she couldn't come with me, but her presence gave me some strength. I was then taken by ambulance for the short ride to the airport. The transition to the small airplane felt surreal, but I was comforted by the nurse who accompanied me. Despite being consumed with terror, I was completely exhausted. Historically, I've never been able to stay awake on a plane, and this time was no different. I was grateful for the escape that sleep provided, and I managed to rest for most of the flight. We landed in Vancouver a few hours later and I was still extremely anxious about what lay ahead.

As soon as I arrived at the hospital, a team of doctors was ready to help me. They already had all my information and sprang into action the moment I was wheeled into a triage space and closed the curtains. One was hooking me up to various machines, another was asking me questions, and another was giving me a thorough examination. It was an extremely overwhelming sensation being surrounded by that many caretakers at once. As I lay back and let them do their jobs, tears gently rolled down my face. I was terrified but at the same time felt a profound sense of safety and reassurance knowing that I was in the best possible place. Hours later, they wheeled me up to my room and finally brought me something to eat. I was absolutely starving! I hadn't been allowed any food in case an emergency surgery was necessary, and my last meal had been dinner the previous evening—well over twenty-four hours ago. The meal they gave me was light but incredibly welcome. With some food in my stomach, I was finally able to relax and rest.

My husband arrived late that night and his presence was the most welcoming sight. It was terrifying being there alone and now to have him there with me was immensely comforting. The hospital staff arranged a small bed for him on the floor next to mine and allowed him to stay with me that first night. Bless their hearts but the floor was cold and uncomfortable for him. The next day he started looking at places nearby that he could stay and found a basement suite that was within walking distance to the hospital. This arrangement ensured he had a comfortable place to sleep and a space to shower. We had no idea how long we were going to be there. Each day was a flurry of activity as my medical team continually monitored my condition, ran tests, and performed ultrasounds to ensure the baby was safe. I walked countless miles up and down the hospital hallways whenever I was allowed to exercise. Each stroll took us past the NICU, where we prayed fervently that we wouldn't have to end up there. The doctors had warned us from the beginning that it was a possibility, but they were doing everything in their power to prevent it.

We had been in the hospital in Vancouver for two weeks when the doctors were convinced they had successfully stopped the labor. They were confident that the baby would carry close to term. I was allowed to return home with strict instructions to rest and take it easy for the remainder of my pregnancy. This meant I wouldn't be going back to work. But after such an incredibly stressful and scary experience, my only concern was the safety of my baby. I wholeheartedly accepted their orders. While we were thrilled to be leaving the hospital and returning home, I couldn't help but feel somewhat apprehensive about leaving the security of such excellent medical care. We still had several weeks to go before the baby would no longer be considered premature and that was unsettling. However, the doctors were reassuring and seemed confident in their prognosis, so I did my best to trust their expertise. We were both excited and ready to get home. I found it strange that medical benefits flew me to the destination, but the return arrangements were at my own expense. We booked our flights for the following day and flew home together. Once we arrived, my husband then had the logistical challenge of retrieving his truck that he had left at an airport two provinces away.

Once I was home and settled, I went to the firehall to submit my medical forms and update them on my status. Nothing ever goes according to plan with a pregnancy and mine was no exception. My initial plan was to work until the last day possible and then take my full maternity leave after the baby was born. But with the recent complications, that plan had changed drastically, and I had to come to terms with it. It was an important reminder for me that this was no longer about my personal goals or desires; it was about ensuring the health and safety of my baby. Consequently, I was placed on medical leave from work for the remainder of my pregnancy. Adjusting to this new reality required me to slow down and prioritize rest, which was a task that proved to be challenging for someone who was accustomed to always being active and on the go. As difficult as it was, I knew this was a temporary situation and the absolute best course of action for both me and my baby.

While I was on medical leave, our city experienced one of the largest fires in the downtown core. A historic hotel and restaurant caught fire. This was the first time it felt incredibly painful for me not to be there to help my team. It was torture knowing it was happening and how tirelessly everyone would be working. I couldn't resist the urge to be present and at least show some support for my colleagues. I made my way to the scene and found a command truck that was blocking traffic to the downtown area. I stood there watching in awe as the fire raged through the buildings and sent plumes of black smoke billowing into the sky. It was a surreal experience to witness such a massive blaze from the outside. Normally, I would have been right in the thick of it, unable to see the scene from this perspective. Just standing there was unbearable as I felt a deep need to contribute somehow. Being extremely mindful of staying out of the smoke and not getting in the way, I grabbed the department's camera from the command truck and started taking pictures from my vantage point. Though I couldn't get any closer, at least capturing the scene allowed me to feel somewhat involved. By no means did it fully satisfy my desire to be part of the action, but at least I felt like I had contributed in a small way.

I was able to carry the baby to full term, and on November 18, 2012, our beautiful, healthy baby boy came earthside via an emergency C-section. Once again, it was the opposite of what I had planned, but by this point I was becoming accustomed to unexpected turns. The arrival of our son was an incredibly exciting time for our family, filled with overwhelming joy and gratitude.

Why had no one explained to me how instantly and profoundly I would love this tiny baby? The intensity of this love was unlike anything I had ever experienced. It was beyond words and immeasurable in its depths. Holding my son for the first time, I was flooded with an array of emotions I didn't even know existed.

Physically, I struggled severely due to the incision and the significant blood loss I endured. Maneuvering myself and fulfilling the tasks required of being a new mother were incredibly challenging. Consequently, much to my displeasure, I had an extended stay in the hospital. Despite the discomfort, I knew it was for the best. I felt immense relief that our son's arrival was safe, and we had made it to his expected due date. Throughout this time, I constantly reminded myself that despite the challenges and deviations from our plans, we were truly blessed with our miracle baby. The joy of his birth outweighed the difficulties, and I was excited for the beginning of a wonderful new chapter in our lives.

The excitement I felt for my son's arrival was unfortunately short-lived as I soon found myself suffering horribly with severe postpartum depression. I visited my doctor to express my concerns, only to be told that what I was experiencing was completely normal and merely the "baby blues." I was assured that I would be fine, to just give it time, and advised to return only if I felt the urge to harm myself or my baby. Having never gone through anything like this before, I trusted my doctor's assessment and internalized the belief that I must be at fault. I blamed myself entirely and thought there was something I was doing wrong. Like every challenge prior to this, I was determined not to appear weak, so I chose to push through it on my own. I convinced myself that sheer willpower would be enough to overcome the overwhelming feelings I was experiencing.

My husband had to return to work shortly after our son was born, which meant I would be left on my own with our son for a few months. The prospect of caring for our newborn by myself terrified the shit out of me, and I truly struggled to cope with the massive responsibility.

"Make sure you keep an eye on him," the nurse said to me when we left the hospital, "because at any time he could stop breathing."

Those words filled me with absolute terror, buried deep within my soul, and played back to me on repeat. As a result, I hardly took my eyes off my son and watched him constantly day and night. I was on my own, and I was not well. The weight of my postpartum depression and the constant vigilance took a heavy toll on my mental and physical health. I was deeply suffering, but I pushed myself to manage because I needed to be strong for my son. The pressure of being solely responsible for his well-being when I felt barely alive myself was immense. Every single day was a struggle to hold myself together while ensuring he was safe and cared for. That was often easier said than done when I had constant thoughts of running away—of getting in my vehicle and driving until I couldn't drive anymore. I would put my son down for a nap and then sit on the stairs and stare out the window at the road, lost in those thoughts. I wondered how I could time it just right so that my mom would arrive before my son was awake—alone. I meticulously contemplated options for how I could disappear without a trace. How I could avoid being tracked through my bank card or my phone. It was serious. Yet each time that I sat there, painstakingly working out all the details, I knew deep down that I couldn't go through with it. The thought of my son waking up alone and scared tore my heart to pieces. I imagined his frightened face and lonely cry, and that was enough to shatter any desire I had to leave. I was desperate, but I couldn't bring myself to do that to him. My strength lay in staying and putting his needs above my own. As badly as I wanted to escape my struggles, I had to be there for my son. Thankfully, his well-being mattered more than my desire to run away, and having enough clarity for that understanding saved me.

My mother, who caught on that I was struggling even though I refused to admit it, was a constant source of support. She made it a point to check in on us daily and her visits were my lifeline. She provided me with practical assistance, emotional support, and the reassurance I desperately needed. She helped with everything from household chores to caring for her grandson, which allowed me time to rest and regain some strength. I hadn't been sleeping and it showed. My mother's unwavering support taught me invaluable lessons about love and motherhood. She showed me that it was okay to accept help and that being strong sometimes meant leaning on others. Her presence made a world of difference and eased the frantic panic of being on my own. I am forever grateful for her guidance and love during those challenging times. Without her, I would have been completely lost and afraid of what I may have succumbed to out of desperation. Her support not only helped me survive that extremely difficult period but also shaped my understanding of unconditional love as a mother.

CHAPTER 16

An Identity Crisis

I was experiencing a severe identity crisis. Over the past few years, I had molded myself to fit into the role of being a firefighter. I never aspired to be "one of the guys," but I had downplayed and hid my feminine side significantly, trying to blend in. I got breast implants years before becoming a firefighter to feel more feminine, but I made it a point to stop wearing clothes that highlighted my figure. I removed anything that could be sexualized in hopes of being taken seriously in a male-dominated field. This adaptation became a core part of who I was.

Now I suddenly found myself stepping into the role of a mother, with no idea how to navigate this new identity. It was completely foreign, yet it was the most important role I would ever assume. The transition from firefighter to mother was severe and I was struggling to balance these two parts of myself.

To some, my concerns might have seemed trivial; to me, they were deeply significant. I was navigating the monumental responsibilities of motherhood, feeling uncertain about how to act and even how to dress. In my mind, becoming a mother meant that I needed to adopt a different demeanor and appearance than I had before. The idea of being a mother brought with it a set of expectations that I struggled to define. I couldn't simply continue doing things the same way I had before; everything felt different now. Even the clothes in my closet seemed inadequate, as if they didn't fit the image of how I believed a mother should dress. Nor did they fit this new body I was sporting. While I couldn't pinpoint exactly what "mom clothes" were supposed to look like, I knew that my current wardrobe did *not* align with this new identity I was embracing.

My husband, bless his heart, couldn't fully understood the depth of my struggle, but he recognized how impactful all these changes were to me. In a gesture of support, he planned a weekend getaway to the city so I could tackle my wardrobe dilemma head-on. Without hesitation, we made the arrangements, packed our bags, and set off the following weekend for my much-needed shopping spree. We arrived in the bustling city and wasted no time diving into the shopping experience. We stepped into a vast clothing store, and I was immediately overwhelmed by the array of choices before me. While I admired the perfectly coordinated outfits on the displays, I was at a loss when it came to assembling a cohesive look for myself. The concept of "mom clothes" suddenly seemed super challenging. My husband saw my frustration and growing sense of despair and sprang into action. Without skipping a beat, he approached the sales counter and inquired about the possibility of enlisting the help of a personal shopper. To my surprise, the store did offer this service, and my husband quickly arranged for me to be paired with one. I instantly wanted to cry. The simple act of seeking assistance from a personal shopper was something I never would have considered doing for myself. If I had been left to my own devices, I likely would have left the store feeling defeated and in tears.

My husband wished me luck, gave me a kiss, and then whisked our son away in the stroller. I remained, ready to embark on a wardrobe transformation with the assistance of a kind-hearted professional. From the moment we began, it was clear that she was more than just an employee; she was an angel sent to guide me through this daunting process. With patience and empathy, she listened attentively as I shared my thoughts and insecurities about my wardrobe and my changing body. Without a hint of judgment, she offered me gentle reassurance and practical advice. Together, we ventured into various parts of the store, where she skillfully selected a few foundational pieces to kickstart my new wardrobe. She got me settled into the dressing room, where I eagerly tried on each garment. She waited outside for the reveal of each piece, then provided additional options and styling suggestions. With her guidance and suggestions, I began to see the potential in mixing and matching pieces to create versatile outfits that fulfilled the vision of my mom style. Each time I emerged from the dressing room adorned in carefully curated ensembles, I couldn't help but feel a newfound sense of confidence and empowerment. These outfits embodied everything I had envisioned mom clothes to be! They were comfortable, practical, yet effortlessly stylish. Thanks to the patient guidance of my personal shopper, I not only found the perfect pieces for my wardrobe, but I also rediscovered a sense of self-assurance and joy in the process.

Two hours later, as I was finishing up in the dressing room, my husband returned. I could hardly contain my excitement as I prepared to show him what I had picked out. For the first time in months, I felt comfortable in my own skin and confident in my new identity as a mother. It was a truly transformative moment, and finally I felt like I was dressed for the part. I showed him the pieces I had selected and saw his face light up with approval. He was genuinely happy and excited for me, which reinforced my newfound confidence.

CHAPTER 17

Motherhood Over My Career

Throughout my pregnancy, my husband and I had many discussions about childcare options, and we concluded there were very limited choices. My husband worked away from home while I worked shift work and was expected to be on call between my shifts. When my pager went off, I had to respond immediately, regardless of the time of day or night. This made it impossible to manage without someone living with us who could provide consistent care for our baby. One option stood out: hire a live-in nanny. Given our small town and northern isolated location, we wouldn't find anyone local to fill the position. So as soon as our son was born, we began the process of hiring a live-in nanny from the Philippines. We knew the process typically took about six months to complete, so that gave us ample time to have her settled in with our family before I returned to work. We were confident that this plan would allow me to balance my demanding job with the responsibilities of motherhood.

However, things didn't go as smoothly as we had hoped. Imagine my surprise and dismay when the process came to an abrupt halt halfway through due to the government temporarily suspending the hiring of migrant workers. This threw our plan into complete disarray, leaving us scrambling for solutions. We corresponded constantly with the nanny agency and a government representative, exploring every possible avenue and loophole we could to expedite the process. But despite our best efforts, it became clear that our nanny's arrival was going to be significantly delayed, potentially extending months beyond the end of my maternity leave. This news was incredibly disheartening. I felt a growing sense of panic. Returning to work without the nanny wasn't an option given my on-call responsibilities and the lack of alternative childcare solutions. The delay placed immense stress on our family as it jeopardized my ability to go back to work and maintain the career I had worked so hard to build.

I explored and exhausted every possible angle—daycares, family, friends, friends of friends, kids of friends, an au pair—but in the end, I came up empty-handed. There were no viable alternatives left, so I was faced with a heart-wrenching sacrifice. I had to resign from my career. The thought alone was devastating. It took me a few days to summon the courage to sit down and type out my resignation letter. My heart felt shattered. This didn't feel real. I had poured my heart and soul into my career and had conquered countless obstacles along the way, but this was one obstacle I couldn't overcome. Now, I had to let it all go. The weight of this decision was almost unbearable. Although I knew without a doubt that my son's well-being was more important than any job, the loss of my career still stung deeply.

When the moment came to drive to the firehall to deliver the resignation letters—one for the union and one for the fire chief—I was an emotional wreck. Tears blurred my vision as I parked and walked into the building. Each step felt heavy with the gravity of my decision. Handing over those envelopes was one of the hardest things I had ever done. It wasn't just about leaving a job; it was about leaving behind a part of myself, a part that had defined me. As I handed the letters to the respective recipients, I had a hard time keeping my composure. They each gave looks of surprise when they read the letter, then questioned if I was sure of my decision. They could see my distress and offered words of support and understanding but it did very little to ease the pain. I explained that this wasn't what I wanted but it was what I had to do.

A short time later, I received an unexpected call from a member of city management. He informed me that he was refusing to accept my resignation and wanted to see me in his office immediately. I drove to City Hall, fully prepared to explain that, despite his refusal, my resignation was unfortunately unavoidable due to my childcare situation. When I arrived, he greeted me with a solemn expression and handed me a box of Kleenex as I sat down. My heart was heavy with the weight of what I had to say. Sharing my struggles out loud was the last thing I wanted to do; everything he needed to know had already been written in my resignation letter. This man had always been one of my greatest supporters and he knew how much effort I had invested to achieve my position. I could see the pain in his eyes as he listened carefully to the justifications of my decision. He wasted no time getting to the point and firmly stated that he wasn't going to allow the lack of childcare to force me out of a career I had worked so hard for. His compassion and understanding overwhelmed me, and I understood how truly valued and important I was to him—which was something that hadn't always come with other leaders on the job. His words filled me with gratitude and a slight glimmer of hope. He reassured me that we were going to find a solution and that he would personally be taking care of the matter and would be in touch soon.

Staying true to his word, a series of meetings were quickly convened, involving the union, fire chiefs, and other city officials. Their collective goal was to find a viable solution that would allow me to remain employed. Unfortunately, they came face-to-face with the same challenges I had encountered and were unable to find any workable answers. However, they were not willing to give up on me, and after much deliberation, it was decided that I would be granted a six-month leave of absence without pay. This would hopefully give us the time we needed to bring our nanny from the Philippines and resolve the childcare issue. While it wasn't a perfect solution, it was a lifeline that allowed me to hold on to my career and hold hope that things would eventually fall into place.

I made sure not to take the additional six months at home with my son for granted. It was truly a blessing in disguise—some days were challenging but having extra time to be present to witness his growth and development was a precious gift. Then, miraculously, one month before my extended leave was set to expire, our live-in nanny arrived. I could finally take a deep exhale of relief. That final month of my leave was dedicated to helping our nanny integrate smoothly into our household and our lives. I introduced her to our family routines, the layout of our home, and the local community. We worked closely together and ensured we all felt comfortable with her new role. This preparation time allowed me to feel secure and confident in her abilities to care for our son and be a member of our family. As my return to work approached, I felt an immense sense of gratitude for the additional time that I had with my son and for the stability of having a trustworthy caregiver and a job to return to.

CHAPTER 18

The Best Of Both Worlds

With reliable childcare in place, I was able to confidently return to work and resume my regular shift schedule. Things felt distinctly different, though it was difficult to pinpoint exactly why. Perhaps it was the sense of purpose and productivity that came from getting out of the house and contributing to my work. Alternatively, it might have been the extended break from a previously toxic environment that allowed me to return feeling rejuvenated. Likely it was a combination of both factors. The break provided me a necessary reset and stepping back into a structured routine reinforced a feeling of normalcy and accomplishment.

During my absence there were some significant changes that had occurred within the department. A few long-time members had retired, and a few new hires had joined the team in their place. Additionally, the annual rotation of crew positions had shifted the workplace dynamics and resulted in a fresh mix of members, which required some adjustment. The atmosphere felt different; there was a noticeable change in the energy of the place. While it wasn't entirely free of toxicity, I could see there was a definite improvement. The overall environment felt more positive, and it brought a smile to my face. It made me hopeful to see some evolution with a diverse mix of personalities and perspectives that could possibly breathe new life into the department, and reflect a shift towards respect, inclusivity, and support—values I've always held close. Again, I was hopeful.

I pulled out my gear bag to go through its contents and get everything set up in my locker as it needed to be. It had been a while since I last touched it. And despite being clean, the bag still carried that familiar, distinctive smell of used fire gear—a mix of smoke, sweat, and ash that represents resilience, survival, and purpose. I had missed that scent. As I unfolded my jacket, something unusual caught my eye. Tucked into a corner of the bag were two neatly folded receiving blankets adorned with fire truck patterns. They were precious! I was curious and touched by the gesture. I looked around, half-expecting to catch sight of whoever might have left them. But the bay was empty; I was alone. With a smile on my face, I picked up the blankets and held them for a moment as I admired the tiny fire trucks on each one. A wave of appreciation washed over me. I had no idea how long they had been there, nor did I ever discover who had left the thoughtful gift.

It took me a while to reacquaint myself with everything and adjust to the new changes that had taken place during my absence. The initial transition back into shift work was a bit challenging, but I soon found my footing. One of the most gratifying aspects of returning was the absence of certain individuals who had previously drained the joy out of both my work and the career I loved. Their retirements felt like a breath of fresh air. Unfortunately, not everything had changed for the better. A few guys remained who hadn't altered their behavior toward me one bit. Although I hadn't considered them as toxic as the ones who had left, their presence was still a challenge. These guys struck me as self-centered, extremely insecure, and manipulative. Unlike their predecessors, they didn't have evil running through their veins but appeared to be driven more by their insecurities and selfish motives. They were reasonably manageable. By avoiding them whenever possible and doing my best to not let their behavior affect me, I could either handle or ignore their antics without too much difficulty.

However, on more than one occasion I would find myself going toe-to-toe with one particular man. He had a habit of getting in my face and making demands, which I did not appreciate. On one instance, he wanted me to approach the chief and accuse him of lying about the gym equipment we had been promised. Since I was on the gym committee, he felt it was my responsibility to confront the chief. But truthfully, I was not in on the private conversation between the chief and the union, so there was no way I was going to take such a stance or make accusations about something I knew nothing about. This guy was relentless in his demands. I moved to various locations in the firehall, trying to distance myself from him, but he followed me to every single one and kept pushing and demanding that I confront the chief. At one point I made my way to the cabinet where our pigeonholes—drawers for keeping letters or documents—were located and hoped that being near the management offices would deter him. I opened the cabinet door and pretended to need something from my drawer. Suddenly he came up right beside me, doing his best to intimidate with his body language. In a quiet but stern voice, he insisted that I do as he said.

Angrily, I turned to face him. "I'm not doing that. If you feel so strongly about it, then you go do it yourself!"

I pushed my drawer in, closed the cabinet, and irritably walked away. He continued to follow me wherever I went. I repeatedly told him to stop and leave me alone, but he ignored my demands for space. Eventually, I had to lock myself in the bathroom just to get away from him.

I flushed the toilet, pretending that I had used it, then ran the water in the sink as if washing my hands, finishing with a wasted piece of paper towel pulled from the dispenser. It was all an act, just to seem like I wasn't hiding. Once I felt I'd stalled long enough, I slowly unlocked and opened the bathroom door. I looked to see if the coast was clear and saw no one. Though I was annoyed, I felt a sense of relief. I headed out into the truck bay and heard voices coming from the far side. I walked across the bay, following the sound of voices. As soon as I turned the corner, I found him conversing with the crew as they cleaned a truck. There were three other firefighters present, but his attention immediately turned to me, and he came at me again. This time, he kept pointing his finger in my face, telling me that he was senior to me, and I had to do as I was told.

"Stop pointing your finger in my face!" I demanded. "That is something I absolutely hate."

He completely ignored my request and continued his demands while pointing his finger. A wave of frustration and resentment surged through me, the sting of being disregarded hitting hard. Fueled by the sheer disrespect my patience had reached its limit and I could feel the anger rising.

I leaned in close and let loose: "Get your fucking finger out of my face before I break it!"

Before he could respond, one of the other firefighters jumped down off the truck and positioned himself between us, facing him. He calmly explained that while he understood the other guy's position of seniority and rank, he also knew that I was a lady, and he couldn't stand by and allow a lady to be disrespected.

"She asked you nicely to stop pointing your finger in her face several times," he cautioned. "You need to stop."

A tense silence followed as they stood face-to-face for a few seconds. Finally, the senior member turned and walked away. I let out a long exhale and realized only then that I had been holding my breath.

I thanked the firefighter for standing up for me and for doing what he did.

He gave me a respectful nod. "I know you're a firefighter. But you're also a lady. I couldn't let him treat a lady like that."

His words were both kind and firm and emphasized the respect he believed I deserved. He then added that payback was probably coming for him. We both knew that was an accurate presumption. It was probably coming for both of us. Challenging someone senior like that, even for good reason, would surely come with consequences. I told him I appreciated his support and understood the risk he took. It didn't go unnoticed that he was the only one willing to step in, and it meant a lot to me.

That was one of the first times I truly felt a sense of power activate within me. Standing my ground and refusing to back down filled me with a pride I hadn't experienced before. Even though there was the potential for repercussions, I felt emboldened by my actions. The possibility that revenge was coming for me at some point was high. The man I had stood up to was in a position of authority, known to be vengeful, and challenging him was not something that would be easily forgiven. Yet in that moment, I realized that my veneration was reserved for the position, not the man who occupied it. His behavior had eroded any personal respect I might have had for him, and standing up to his bullying had felt both necessary and right.

Overall, it felt great to be back at work, active in the job I loved, having adult conversations, and challenging my mind and body again. One of the aspects I cherished most was the constant variety. Each day brought something new: different training sessions, varied chores, and unpredictable calls. The uncertainty of when an emergency would arise or what it would entail was something I thrived on. Don't get me wrong, I loved being a mother. But it felt stifling being at home, where every day followed the same routine. I thrived on change and challenge. Even back when I was a hairstylist, the diversity of my clients and their hairstyles kept me on my toes. Each client was unique and required creativity, risk-taking, and physical endurance. Being a firefighter offered a similar dynamic in that every day presented new situations that demanded quick thinking and decisive action.

Returning to work reignited a spark in me that had been dimmed for a while. Although motherhood carried its own sense of purpose and value, I yearned to fulfill more than one mission: motherhood and career. I am someone who needs to—and has the energy for—working on my full purpose. I didn't want to compartmentalize and shut off valuable offerings I know I bring to my family, my community, and my work. Admitting this to myself was difficult and I carried extreme guilt about longing to return to work for a long time. The societal expectations and unsolicited opinions from others only compounded that guilt. People were always quick to share their thoughts about my choices, and their opinions weren't helpful. But I grew accustomed to their judgment and the commentary. I had always lived a bit outside of the norm, and that seemed to provoke some and inspire others. The truth was, I thrived on the challenges and unpredictability of my job. Being at home, where every day felt like a repetition of the last, stifled me. I needed the dynamic environment of work to feel alive and engaged. This wasn't to say that I didn't love my family or cherish my time with my son, but my fulfillment came from a balance of home life and the stimulating demands of my career.

I felt incredibly grateful to have the best of both worlds. I could immerse myself in my work and fulfill that part of me that thrived there, then come home to be a mother and embrace the love and joy that family life brought me. This balance was only possible because of our amazing nanny, who cared for our son as if he were her own and managed our home with extraordinary skill and dedication. She went above and beyond for our family and attended to every detail with grace and understanding. Her ability to fill in for me was invaluable. Knowing that our son and our home was in such capable hands allowed me to easily have both a professional and a personal life. It was a rare and precious balance I knew I was fortunate to possess but the pressures I faced ultimately overshadowed that sense of security and would profoundly impact us both in our journey.

My pager would go off at any given time and pull me away for unpredictable periods, depending on the call. I could be gone for an hour for a minor incident or twelve-plus hours for a major emergency. I didn't realize how much pressure I placed on myself and how it was affecting me during that first year back at work. The constant uncertainty and the need for everything to run smoothly at home made me extremely controlling and demanding. I wanted to ensure that every aspect of my home life was meticulously managed so that I could focus entirely on my work when I was there without distractions or worries.

Over the past few years, I had been trapped in a cycle of fear at work, feeling powerless against the words and actions directed at me. This lack of control over my circumstances left me grasping for control in other areas of my life, particularly in my relationships with those I trusted. In my quest for security, I placed unrealistic expectations on myself and my loved ones. I believed that control equaled safety, so I became a fervent micromanager who dictated every detail of my environment to ward off any potential threats. My need for control stemmed from my sense of powerlessness in the face of men in authority positions in my workplace. Since I was unable to assert myself in that realm, I compensated for it by exerting dominance in my personal space and against those I loved.

There was a toll for this constant battle for control and it manifested in my demeanor. I was tense, irritable, and quick to anger, especially toward the nanny, even though she was an invaluable support in managing the chaos of my life. Unfortunately, she fell victim to my relentless need for control. I scrutinized her every move as if I didn't trust her to uphold the standards I imposed. I had made my job at the firehall a priority, and it came before everyone's needs, including my own. This single-minded focus came at the expense of genuine connection with those around me. A pivotal period for me was understanding that my behavior was driven by fear, insecurity, and unhealed wounds. I was living in a trauma response. It was painful to acknowledge the ways in which I took our nanny for granted and failed to truly appreciate her dedication, support, and kindness. I was unable to accept or reciprocate her love and she deserved so much better than the emotional distance I maintained.

Achieving a balance between my career and family life required significant suffering and sacrifice on multiple fronts. The nature of my shift work did offer some advantages, as I was only away from my son for two day shifts. During my two night shifts, he was mostly asleep. I would then have four consecutive days off that provided valuable time to reconnect with my family. However, the constant presence of my pager tethered me to my professional duties and was the biggest pain in the ass for everyone. My pager would often interrupt family gatherings, birthday parties, grocery shopping, and even cherished holidays like Christmas morning. When it went off, I had no choice but to drop everything and respond immediately. I would leave my family to go and attend to someone else's needs. This duality of being a caregiver to my own family and a responder to the needs of the community was both a blessing and a curse. On one hand, I felt a deep sense of purpose in being able to provide support and assistance during someone else's time of need. But this came at the cost of missing out on precious moments and milestones with my loved ones. It also came at the cost of the nanny's life being placed in a holding pattern in case I needed her.

My family understood the importance of my work and me being grounded in the service of others. While it was often difficult to reconcile the moments of regret for sacrifices my loved ones made, I did take solace in knowing that my efforts made a meaningful difference in the lives of those I served. It was a constant juggling act, but it was one that I approached dutifully.

CHAPTER 19

I Was A Role Model

I considered myself truly fortunate to have the opportunity to serve my community in a manner that no one else had before. As the first ever and only female in my position, I recognized the unique advantage and responsibility that came with it. It was a privilege bestowed upon me, and one that I didn't take lightly. Being a trailblazer in my field allowed me to break barriers and challenge stereotypes. I was personally entrusted with the task of demonstrating to people, particularly young individuals, what was achievable regardless of gender. It was a role that I embraced wholeheartedly, and I understood the impact it could have on shaping perceptions and inspiring future generations.

Wearing my firefighter uniform was a symbol of honor, opportunity, and inspiration. One of the greatest privileges of donning that uniform and being present within the community was the chance to interact with children and ignite their enthusiasm for a career that I considered to be the coolest job in the world—firefighting. This was especially true for little girls. I relished the opportunity to educate and encourage young minds and show them that firefighting wasn't only a career for boys. The joy and excitement I saw in their eyes upon realizing that girls could be firefighters too, were truly heartwarming. It was a moment of realization that transcended the pages of books or the scenes on television. Right before them stood a living, breathing, walking, talking, girl firefighter. I was someone who defied stereotypes and shattered preconceived notions. Getting to witness the spark of possibility that ignited within these children was nothing short of magical. I watched as their imaginations soared as they explored avenues and dreams that they might not have considered before. It was a privilege to be a part of that transformative moment, and to plant the seeds of ambition and empowerment in their young minds. As I stood before these children, I knew I was embodying a beacon of hope and was a testament to the boundless possibilities that awaited them.

These young minds overflowing with wonder sparked the most genuine and vibrant questions and comments. Sometimes their curiosity led to moments that tested my composure as their innocent inquiries veered into unexpected territory. Other times, their words struck a chord deep within me and touched on personal experiences that they felt safe enough to share. These interactions were a delicate balance between maintaining a professional demeanor and allowing myself to be moved by their sincerity. During each exchange, I was acutely aware of the honor and privilege that was bestowed upon me. The opportunity to make a positive impact on these little lives by inspiring, encouraging, and instilling confidence in them was a privilege I cherished deeply.

I got some interesting—and often humorous—questions and comments from kids:

"Aren't you scared?"

"Can you wear a dress with your gear on?"

"Why are you the only girl here? There should be all girls!"

"The fire truck is *so* big. How can you drive it? My mom backed our motorhome into a tree."

"If there is a fire at my house, will you come and save me?"

"I want to be a firefighter so I can start fires and then put them out."

"My dad called you when my cat was stuck in a tree, and you wouldn't come rescue him. My dad said it could have died!"

"One time our house caught on fire, and my mom had to run back into the fire to get some important things because we didn't have any money to get new ones. She burned her feet because she didn't have any shoes on."

"Firefighters are way cooler than police."

And the one that I treasure the most and hold near and dear to my heart: "I want to be a firefighter just like you!"

I was a role model, and I never took my position for granted. Every chance I had to share, speak, educate, and encourage, I seized with enthusiasm. The positive feedback I received from parents was a testament to the impact I was making. Parents often told me how their children—even the quietest ones who had watched me with hesitation—went home brimming with exciting stories about meeting a girl firefighter. Their newfound enthusiasm made me smile because I had connected with them. Whether they learned a fire safety tip or dreamed of becoming firefighters themselves, I knew I had done my job. The moments of connection were countless and precious. I will forever cherish the hugs, the heartfelt "I love you's," the enthusiastic high fives, and the looks of adoration I received from those young faces. Each interaction held a special place in my heart and served as a reminder of the significance of my role. It wasn't just about imparting knowledge or sparking career aspirations; it was about being a tangible example of possibility. Every classroom visit, and every firehall tour became an opportunity to break down barriers and show these children that they could achieve anything they set their minds to. Seeing their eyes light up with understanding and inspiration was a reward beyond measure. I felt a deep sense of fulfillment knowing that I was not only teaching important safety skills but also expanding their horizons and instilling confidence. I was grateful for every single moment, and they fueled my passion for my work. I will carry those memories with me and my hope is that I made a lasting, positive influence on those young lives.

My role modeling extended beyond the public sphere, as I had an eager pair of eyes and ears at home. My son adored everything about the fire trucks, the fire department, and his firefighter mother. His enthusiasm was boundless. He had his own miniature set of gear, including a special helmet at the firehall that one of my colleagues lent him and allowed him to call his own. From the time he was two he knew the names of every truck and could barely contain his excitement whenever we passed the firehall. I couldn't drive by without stopping in because he always wanted to sit in the trucks and chat with the firefighters.

He knew his way around the firehall and always made sure he paid a visit to every crew member and every office. Even at his young age, he understood the dynamics of the fire department. He knew that while I was his mother, I wasn't the one in charge there. He always showed great respect for the chain of command and politely asked the captain on duty for permission before exploring the trucks. Every visit became a learning adventure. I would explain the intricacies of the fire engines, how the equipment worked, and the importance of each tool. My son absorbed it all with wide-eyed fascination. I would watch him immerse himself in his role-playing, pretending to be a firefighter driving the trucks, and it was a source of endless joy for me. His curiosity and eagerness to learn reminded me why I loved my job so much. It wasn't just about fighting fires; it was about educating and inspiring others, especially the next generation.

As my son made his rounds to everyone, he couldn't quite pronounce some of their names correctly, being so young. But his attempts brought immense joy to everyone he encountered. He confidently greeted the deputy chief with a hearty, "Hi, Depurly," then shook his hand with the earnestness only a child could muster. The broad smile that spread across the deputy chief's face warmed my heart every time. The nickname Depurly became a cherished part of our lives, and the deputy chief graciously accepted it, and allowed me to use it as well. For some of the others, my son combined their names and created his own. These moments were more than just adorable interactions; they were solid connections that underscored the community and camaraderie that my son and I were privileged to be part of. He was as much a part of the department as I was, having forged strong relationships with the good men there—men who I knew would do anything for him and treated him like family.

Seeing my son's eyes light up with fascination and pride whenever we visited the firehall was a reminder of the importance of my role not just as a firefighter, but as a mother and a role model. His excitement and confidence in what I had chosen as a career made every sacrifice and challenge feel worthwhile. These experiences at the firehall also strengthened our bond. They allowed us to share a part of my world that was crucial to my identity, and it meant the world that he was proud of who his mother was and what she did for a living. I cherished these interactions and hoped that they were laying the foundation for my son to grow up with a strong belief that he could achieve anything he set his mind to.

For my son's fourth birthday, I arranged a photoshoot at the firehall because he wanted a firefighter-themed celebration. He was ecstatic, all dressed up in his miniature firefighter gear, and ready to pose with "his crew." My colleagues were supportive and kind and put on their turnout gear and joined us for some of the photos. Their willingness to participate added a special touch to the occasion and made it even more memorable. There was immense pride in my son's eyes as he stood as a firefighter alongside us. It wasn't just a birthday-themed photoshoot; it was a moment of connection and shared joy. The guys on my crew mirrored his pride and were happy to be part of such a special day for him. It was a heartwarming sight to see my little boy brimming with excitement as he methodically chose which trucks to pose with and decided on the perfect stances for each photo. Each snapshot captured the fulfilment of a young boy's dream and a precious moment in time.

CHAPTER 20

The Same But Different

I have always been physically fit, even long before I became a firefighter. From an early age, I cultivated a strong and muscular physique through dedicated training and an active lifestyle. Fitness has always been a core part of who I am. However, when I joined the fire department, the importance of my physical fitness took on a whole new dimension. Becoming a firefighter meant that my training needed to evolve to meet the unique demands of the job. It was no longer just about building muscle or enhancing endurance; it required a careful balance between the two. The nature of firefighting demands both strength and stamina, often in extreme and prolonged situations. I needed to have the power to lift heavy equipment and the endurance to sustain that power over extended periods.

Finding this balance was initially challenging. If I focused too much on building muscle, I found that my endurance suffered, which is crucial for tasks like climbing multiple flights of stairs with gear or conducting extended rescue operations. Conversely, if I concentrated too much on endurance training, then I began to lose the muscle mass and strength that was necessary to handle the physical rigors of the job effectively.

Through a process of trial and error, I learned to harmonize these two aspects of fitness. I integrated a diverse training regimen that included weightlifting for strength, cardiovascular exercises for endurance, and functional workouts that mimicked the real-life demands of firefighting. This holistic approach allowed me to build a physique that was not only strong and muscular but also highly resilient and capable of enduring the toughest situations. Mastering this balance was a significant achievement.

Being a woman in a predominantly male profession meant that I had to approach certain tasks differently. Physically, I was obviously built differently than the guys, which meant I needed to adapt my techniques to perform the same tasks effectively. While I could achieve the same results, my methods sometimes had to differ due to our physical differences. In the beginning, this approach led to some friction. There was a prevailing expectation that I should perform tasks in the exact same manner as my male colleagues. Some even went so far as to suggest that if I couldn't meet these expectations, I shouldn't be a firefighter. They struggled to understand that different techniques could yield the same effective outcomes. To navigate this challenge, I often found myself having to compromise. When working with certain guys, I would start tasks the way they expected, ensuring that I met their initial approval. But as soon as their attention shifted, I would adjust my positioning or technique to align with what worked best for me.

I didn't have the same upper body strength as most of the men, so holding a large, charged hose line alone for any length of time was particularly exhausting. More often than not, I would be on a hose line without backup. So instead of quickly fatiguing my arm muscles, I developed a technique that utilized my body's strengths more effectively. I would place the hose between my legs, stagger my stance, and squeeze with my thighs to take the pressure off my arms. This method worked amazingly well. By doing this, I could stand at the end of a charged 2.5" line and spray water solo for extended periods.

"What the fuck are you doing?" was a question I often heard about my technique. Followed by an eye roll or a head shake.

Sometimes I was made fun of with comments about liking the feel of a hose between my legs, but I considered the remarks childish and brushed them off. What mattered most was that the technique worked for me and enabled me to get the job done without compromising my physical well-being.

I was also very flexible and could fit into much smaller spaces than most of my male colleagues. This ability proved invaluable in various situations, such as crawling into the confined spaces of a motor vehicle to extricate a patient or maneuvering through a small window for entry or exit during an emergency. I believed it was crucial to have a diverse range of strengths within the department. Each of us brought unique abilities to the team. There would always be tasks that my colleagues could perform that I couldn't and vice versa. While I might not have had the brute strength that some of the men possessed, I had a unique knack for capturing a patient's attention and ensuring they followed commands. The same rang true with children in medical emergencies or traumatic motor vehicle incidents—I evoked a maternal trust that created a sense of safety. I always thought it was our diverse set of skills and the way we complemented each other's strengths and weaknesses that made our team truly effective.

There were undoubtedly many things that set me apart from others in the department, but one issue stood out prominently: being a woman and having to wear men's clothing. I was employed for six years before I finally received a uniform designed for a woman. The only exception occurred when I became pregnant, forcing the department to order a maternity uniform for me. However, before and after that, they consistently refused to provide me with a woman's uniform, insisting instead that I wear men's clothing and get them altered if needed. The individual who took care of the clothing orders every year insisted that all orders were exclusively for men and refused to make an exception for just one person. On multiple occasions I highlighted the indifference and asked for proper clothing but was told that it wasn't a significant issue.

"It's not a fashion show, Lynnette," I was told. "No one cares that the crotch of your pants doesn't fit. They're usually covered by your turnout gear anyways."

I cared, and this dismissal of my needs was extremely frustrating and disheartening. I often imagined the outrage that would have ensued if the roles were reversed, and the men were required to wear women's uniforms simply because it was deemed the only option and "not a big deal."

To me, the uniform was more than just clothing; it signified a sense of professionalism. I understood it wasn't a fashion show, but I also believed that when a person looks the part, they feel the part. Unfortunately, every year I had to take my uniform pants to a seamstress for alterations because they didn't fit properly—for obvious reasons. This was not only inconvenient but also an extra cost and effort that seemed unwarranted. Each year, I would politely ask my colleague, who was responsible for ordering, to get women's pants for me, and even emphasized how it would save both time and money. But despite my persistent requests, the answer was always a resounding no, followed by a long explanation of complete bullshit justifications for sticking to the bulk orders of only men's clothing. In desperation, I even asked for the company's contact information so I could request a women's catalogue and pay for the pants myself. However, the union quickly proclaimed this as not an option as it was contractual, and we were forbidden to deviate outside of the contract. Through the frustration and defeat, every year I voiced my desires.

After six long years of wearing ill-fitting pants and shirts that fit like gunny sacks, I was shocked when the powers that be finally listened to my repeated requests and ordered women's uniform cargo pants and a fitted dress shirt for me. While the unisex T-shirts had never been an issue, having a properly fitting uniform marked a significant shift in my sense of identity and professionalism. I'm not sure what prompted their change of heart, and I never did ask. I was simply grateful for it and welcomed the improvement in my work attire.

It was the same story with my turnout gear. Initially, all the gear was of one style, and it fit in all the worst ways. The poor fit made it extremely hard to work in and left hazardous spaces, increasing the risk of burns. Eventually, we were each measured for more fitted gear, but even then, it didn't fit me quite right. It was significantly better than before, so I was thankful and welcomed the new gear with excitement.

Two years before I retired, I was scheduled to receive new turnout gear as mine was expiring. The manufacturer had just announced that women's turnout gear was now available in Canada. To say I was excited was an understatement! I was measured for a custom set of women's turnout gear and was told by the distributor that it was the very first set made in Canada. I felt incredibly privileged to have the opportunity to finally wear gear designed specifically for my body. When the new turnout gear arrived, I tore open the package like it was a long-awaited gift. I immediately donned it, eager to feel the difference. To my delight, it fit like a glove! The transformation was astounding. It fit correctly and covered all the right places, significantly enhancing my sense of safety and security. It made me realize how much I had been compromising my safety and the risks that had been taken with ill-fitting equipment were, in hindsight, completely unacceptable.

CHAPTER 21

Good Misunderstood

A union executive member was consistently discouraging us firefighters with claims that the public disliked us because they believed we were overpaid and underworked. He argued that we needed to be overly cautious in protecting our image—even going so far as declining support for a basketball net, saying we shouldn't be seen outside exercising. I wholeheartedly disagreed with this perspective and never felt that the community shared such sentiments. On the contrary, I always sensed a strong appreciation and respect from most of the public. I frequently received calls and messages that reinforced this positive perception. Over the years, I worked diligently to build a good rapport within my city, and I firmly believed that I had succeeded in doing so. I often wondered if the one doing the discouraging was projecting his own insecurities onto the rest of us and using his own personal experiences of being disliked by generalizing the entire community's attitude. The many conversations I had with business owners, residents, and even individuals who I assisted during emergencies consistently reflected a high level of satisfaction and gratitude for our services. They regularly praised the professional conduct and dedication of our department members. Their feedback made me proud to be part of the team and confident in the positive impact we had on the community.

One area I was particularly passionate about educating the public on was car seat safety. I was dedicated to ensuring that young children were as safe as possible while traveling. Having responded to numerous motor vehicle incidents involving children, I had witnessed firsthand the life-saving benefits of properly installed and correctly used car seats. Conversely, I had also seen the heartbreaking consequences when these safety measures were neglected. Educating myself about car seat safety became a top priority, and I made it my mission to spread awareness and knowledge to friends, family, and the wider community.

With the changing seasons, I wanted to be proactive in raising awareness about winter car seat safety. I believed this to be important topic because bulky winter clothes, like puffy jackets or snowsuits can create a gap between the child and the car seat harness, reducing its effectiveness in a crash. To achieve this awareness, I sought permission to organize a car seat check event where community members could come to the firehall and have their car seats inspected and receive education pertaining to their seat's usage during the colder months. My bosses loved the idea, my request was approved, and a full-day event was scheduled. I was excited and wanted to promote it, so I made a personal post on my Facebook page, inviting my friends and encouraging them to visit the firehall for the event. By addressing my post to those I knew and cared about, I hoped to ensure their children's safety along with fostering a community-wide culture of car seat awareness.

Shortly after the event was announced, a union executive member confronted me in the upstairs hallway at the firehall and accused me of being selfish and not a team player. He claimed that, as a low-ranking member, I had no right to create such an event without proper authorization.

"I did discuss it with my captain first and he thought it was a great idea!" I scrambled to explain. "He told me to bring it to the chiefs for their approval, so that's what I did."

Even after I explained everything, he continued to insist that I was out of line.

"You have upset everyone in the department. Even the wives," he said. "They read your post on Facebook and are wondering why it has to be all about you. Why are their firefighters excluded? It's selfish."

My heart was racing! Their spouses? I was struggling to understand. They were reportedly upset that I had invited people to "come down and see *me*" rather than framing the event as a departmental initiative. This group reaction took me by surprise because I had intended the post to be a personal invitation to *my* friends, who I believed would feel more comfortable attending if they knew a familiar face would be there. Feeling blindsided, I couldn't comprehend how this had turned into something so negative, and I caught myself questioning my own wording and what I had done wrong. I desperately tried to explain my true intentions.

"I didn't mean to exclude anyone or make it all about me," I emphasized. "I was just trying to encourage my friends to participate."

But even with my best efforts to clarify, I remained deeply hurt by the accusations and the realization that my character was being questioned behind my back. It was devastating to think that others were upset with me. One of my worst fears was coming to life.

I was so overwhelmed by the confrontation that I couldn't speak anymore. I had to walk away as the tears streamed down my face. I locked myself in the bathroom and sank to the floor, struggling to catch my breath. It felt as if the air had been squeezed out of my lungs and the tightness in my chest was excruciating. As I sat there, I replayed his harsh words over and over in my mind and was unable to comprehend how things had escalated to this point. I was confused and hurt. The accusations felt like a betrayal that struck at the core of my intentions and integrity. I had only wanted to help ensure the safety of children in our community, yet my efforts had been completely misconstrued and criticized. The depth of my emotional turmoil felt unbearable, and I couldn't fathom how my genuine intentions got me here.

After some time, I had regained enough composure that I felt comfortable leaving the bathroom. Everyone was at the firehall and preparing to go out into the community for our annual muscular dystrophy boot drive. This was an event I always enjoyed being a part of because it allowed me to engage with the public and make huge contributions to our fundraising efforts. I was determined to keep what had transpired a secret so I could partake in the event without anyone being the wiser. I checked my puffy face in the mirror, took a deep breath and exited the bathroom—only to come face-to-face with the very man I had escaped from to begin with. He had been waiting for me and immediately resumed talking. I snapped! I couldn't take any more of his nonsense. Anger was now surging through me, and I couldn't hold back the tears of rage.

"Shut the fuck up and get away from me!" I screamed. "I don't want to hear anymore!"

He was back peddling and scrambling for words, while trying to block my path in the hallway. All I could think was that I had to leave. I was furious and needed to get the fuck out of there immediately. I told him I was leaving, and again he tried to stop me. Rage burned on my face. He then raised both hands attempting to calm the mess he had created. But I was way beyond reasoning and utterly fed up. I stormed down the stairs and exited through the front door, with him following close behind, still trying to talk to me. I was no longer interested in listening to anything he had to say and couldn't get out of there fast enough.

As I turned the corner, I hesitated. To reach my vehicle, I had to cross the ramp in front of the truck bays. The doors were now open, and the other firefighters were gathered and getting ready to pull the trucks out for the event. There was no way around them. I kept my gaze forward and quickened my pace, trying to move out of sight as fast as possible.

"Where are you going?" my colleagues shouted. "We're leaving! Hurry up!"

I ignored them and focused on reaching the safety of my vehicle. Crossing the ramp felt like the length of a football field. I finally got to my vehicle and jumped in, started the engine, and drove off. I headed straight home, feeling consumed with anger and humiliation.

I couldn't contain my emotions and was sobbing uncontrollably when I walked through the door. My husband was not only surprised to see me, as I was expected to be away for a few hours but was completely shocked by my disheveled state as he watched me struggle to take off my station boots. He immediately reached out for me.

"What's wrong?" he asked.

The moment I felt his arms around me, I collapsed into them, gasping for air between sobs and unable to speak. I was crying so hard I was hyperventilating. I could see the fear and concern in his eyes as he held me and was desperately searching for answers and trying to understand what had happened. The intensity of my emotions had taken over and left me unable to articulate the pain and frustration that had built up inside me. My husband's embrace was the only thing anchoring me in that moment, offering comfort amidst the excruciating turmoil I was experiencing.

It took a few moments before I could gather enough air to speak. Between short, labored breaths, I explained what had happened and how I had been treated. He listened and comforted me, but I could see the anger and frustration in his eyes. I was feeling dizzy and exhausted and needed to lie down. He helped me upstairs to our bedroom and tucked me in. I lay there and cried for a while before finally falling asleep. I was out for a couple of hours, and when I woke, I was disoriented and had a splitting headache. It felt like I had woken from a nightmare, and I wished it *had* been a bad dream. Everything I had worked so hard for, all the good I had tried to do, now felt pointless. It seemed as if everyone had the wrong impression and was angry with me. The mental anguish was too much, and my mind was racing with questions. How the fuck was I going to do damage control on the chaos? Should I just cancel the event so there would be nothing left to be mad about? I was desperately wracking my brain for a solution and concluded that the public deserved for the event to go on. It was for them; it wasn't for us. I decided to change my Facebook post to remove any hint of selfishness. Maybe if the wives saw that I had corrected it and included everyone, then they wouldn't be mad at me anymore. I edited my post and transformed it into a generic invitation that emphasized "us" rather than "me." I carefully removed any personal references and curated the message to reflect the collective effort of the department. I prayed this gesture would demonstrate my commitment to being a team player and would appease everyone who it had upset. The weight of the situation still hung heavily on me, but I hoped this change would help mend the rift and show that my intentions were always for the greater good.

That afternoon, I helped my husband get ready to head back to school. He was home only on weekends and attended school during the week a couple of hours away. As he packed his things, he gave me words of encouragement and tried his best to lift my spirits. We said our goodbyes, and as I watched him drive off, I felt a pang of loneliness. Now it was my turn to get organized and ready because I was transitioning to the night shift. I spent some quality time and cherished moments with my son before saying my goodbyes to him and the nanny. I was putting out intentional effort to stay positive, but a sense of dread settled over me as I prepared to head to work. The thought of returning to the firehall was daunting and I didn't want to face any questions about why I had left earlier and abandoned my position in the boot drive. Driving to work, my mind was a whirlwind of thoughts and apprehension. I didn't want to explain my abrupt departure or the emotional breakdown that had followed. I feared the judgment and misunderstanding that was likely awaiting me. I parked and approached the firehall door, stopping for a moment to take a deep breath before entering the key code. When that door opened, I knew I had to face whatever came next with as much calmness and composure as I could muster.

I began my shift by successfully dodging everyone during the shift change. I immersed myself in various chores and then retreated to the truck bays to tinker with the equipment. Not long after, my captain approached me with the news that two union executive members were on their way to the firehall to speak with me. I immediately assumed this visit was about the incident from that morning and I hoped my decision to amend my Facebook post had been noted and appreciated. Maybe I would even receive an apology. But when the union executives arrived, I quickly learned that their visit was about something entirely different from what I had anticipated.

My phone was set to vibrate and was buzzing incessantly in my pocket. I was standing in the truck bays with my captain and two union executives and was unable to answer the call. One of the executives began describing an unsettling encounter where he had arrived home after work that day to find my husband waiting for him outside of his house. This didn't sound right to me because my husband had left town a few hours earlier to return to school, so I was questioning his story. He insisted that it was him and described how, when he opened his truck door, he was immediately confronted by my visibly upset husband. His voice was trembling, and his hands were noticeably shaking as he recounted the threat my husband had made. He described how my husband was clearly angry about how I had been treated and vowed to return and deal with him if the mistreatment continued. After ensuring his message was understood, my husband walked back to his truck and drove away.

In that moment it hit me: this man had just experienced a complete role reversal. He was the one who had previously confronted me inappropriately—following me around, invading my personal space, making demands and pointing his finger in my face. I wanted to ask him if he now understood how intimidating it felt to be cornered by a man like my husband, the same fear and dread I had endured. How did he like it? Because I never did.

Through this conversation my phone continued to vibrate furiously in my pocket, and I now realized it had to be my husband trying to reach me.

The conversation deepened as it was acknowledged that my husband had targeted the wrong man. The person who had confronted me earlier that morning was not the one my husband had pursued. He was correct in that he had not been directly involved in the altercation. He continued by firmly asserting that my husband's actions were unacceptable and would not be tolerated. How ironic. Frustration mounted within me as, once again, the narrative shifted, and he was casting himself as the victim.

"I'm too old to get in a fight," he expressed. "And I don't stand a chance against your husband."

That was the first honest thing I had ever heard him say! Then he started hinting at involving the authorities and threatening to file a report and possibly press charges. Anger surged through me at his veiled intimidation. I nodded my head in agreement.

"I agree. I think you should go to the police," I calmly confirmed.

He hesitated, looking surprised and slightly bewildered by my response. I seized the moment. "You should definitely go and tell them your version of the event because then I will have the opportunity to go and tell them mine. I will finally get to tell my story and speak my truth, the *whole* truth!"

I continued that not only was I no longer willing to tolerate the harassment, the bullying, and the misogyny, but neither was my family. Everyone's patience had expired, making this the perfect opportunity to unveil the whole truth.

All three men—my captain and the two executive members—questioned me about what "story" I had to tell. The first thing that came to mind was my very first day on the job and the threat I received that I was on my own. I told them outright that I would start with that tidbit and assured them that there was plenty more where that came from. My statement was met with surprise and confusion. They seemed unaware of the threats I had faced on my first day. But as I continued, recounting the backroom meetings I knew had taken place to prevent my hiring, their expressions shifted. All eyes went to the floor. They knew exactly what I was talking about because they had been part of those meetings. The air in the room grew tense with the unspoken truths hanging heavily between us. They were well aware of the lengths they had gone to in their attempts to undermine me and now they were being confronted with the reality of my story and could no longer hide their complicity.

Right before my eyes I watched their attitudes change and the back peddling start almost instantly. The man who had initially insisted we go to the police was now shifting to the suggestion that we should keep what happened a secret between the four of us. He felt that it was in everyone's best interest, particularly mine, to avoid involving the authorities. He claimed he didn't want to get my husband in trouble and implied that protecting him was somehow for my benefit.

Now that he realized the situation was more complex and the battle had become two-sided, he was quick to retreat from his initial stance. I had to stifle a silent chuckle at how easily he had backtracked and was now trying to frame his cowardice as concern for me. My mind was buzzing with all sorts of dialogue about what I truly thought of his sudden change of heart and flimsy excuse, but I kept them to myself. I nodded in agreement only to mask my true intentions. There was no way I would keep what happened a secret anymore! His empty threats, manipulation, and quick cover-up for his own convenience disgusted me.

I addressed them directly. "Every single one of you have wives and daughters, and I would hope to God that if any of them came home in the condition that I did, that you would have the guts to do exactly what my husband did," I stated. "No woman deserves to be treated the way you all have treated me."

I had to throw it back at them in a frame they would hopefully understand. Their responses were muted. I wish I could say they hung their heads in shame, but they didn't. A few moments went by, and they had very little to say in defense because they knew I was right, and their reluctant mutterings confirmed it. I made it very clear that they could not ignore the justice and moral imperative of my stance. That ended our conversation, and we parted ways. I quickly found a quiet spot in a far corner to check my phone, which had finally stopped buzzing in my pocket only moments ago. I pulled it out and saw multiple missed calls, voicemails, and text messages—all from my husband. Without checking any of them, I called him back.

"What did you do?" I blurted out as soon as he answered.

He quickly followed my question with a question.

"Did you get in trouble?" he asked.

I assured him that I didn't and again asked him what he had done. He took a deep breath before he started explaining. He told me that he had always stayed out of anything to do with my job or coworkers because he respected that I was a firefighter before he met me and believed I could handle things myself. And if I couldn't, then it was up to me to figure it out, not him. So he had always left me to deal with everything that happened at work, but this time was different. Seeing the state I was in when I came home had broken him. He couldn't sit back and allow his wife to be treated that way, so he stepped in and did something about it.

I asked why he had gone to that particular guy.

"When you want something done and you want to be heard, you don't fuck around. You go straight to the top," he replied matter-of-factly.

The man he had confronted was at the top, and my husband was heard, so he wasn't wrong. He figured something was going down because I wasn't answering my phone, and he was getting worried, and even considered driving back to check on me. I filled him in on everything that had happened and what was said during my confrontation with the men. I told him how the one he had confronted had threatened to go to the police and press charges, but when I agreed so I could tell my story too, he then changed his tune. His final solution was that we keep things a secret. My husband listened intently as I recounted the rest of what went down. We talked a little more, but I had to get off the phone and back to work since I was technically on the clock.

I considered my husband's actions to be chivalrous and I felt boldly proud of him. As a woman, I could only use my words to get my point across with those men. Often, this could be dismissed as nagging, being a bitch, or I simply wouldn't be heard at all. Men, however, handle things differently and can be known to occasionally settle matters physically. I had seen this firsthand a few times at the firehall. Their aggressive tone isn't taken as nagging; instead, they tend to be heard and taken seriously by other men. I don't believe that I could have ever achieved the result my husband did. His intervention was direct and forceful in a way that commanded respect. When he spoke, he was heard. He has a large presence; therefore, his message was received loud and clear.

In the following days, there were multiple conversations with those involved about what had happened, and I did receive apologies. I took them at face value because I was unsure if they were genuine or driven by fear. Regardless of their motivation, I accepted the apologies, and we agreed to move on. However, I didn't keep what happened a secret between the four of us. My other crew members were curious about the context of the private meeting they had been excluded from that night, so I told them. I believed in transparency and felt that they had a right to know what had transpired. It wasn't something I considered secret-worthy, and it was my story to tell, so I shared it.

I went ahead with the car seat event at the firehall, and it turned out to be a huge success. There was a large number of moms-to-be, new moms, seasoned moms, and even grandparents who came to have their car seats checked and receive important safety education. I was passionate about the message I delivered and the importance of helping people keep their little ones as safe as possible.

As for the issue with the wives being upset with me, I never did find out if there was any truth to the story or get confirmation that changing my Facebook post had smoothed things over. None of them ever approached me directly and the original messenger never brought it up again. The issue quietly faded away. At the end of the day, the purpose of the event was accomplished and that was what mattered the most to me. The satisfaction of knowing a positive impact was made overshadowed any lingering concerns. The rest was just one more thing that got swept under the rug and suppressed.

CHAPTER 22

Disillusionment

For the next few years, work remained largely the same. However, my home life underwent significant changes. Our nanny's three-year contract ended, and she moved on. My husband, now a power engineer, had a rotating shift schedule—one week on, one week off—alternating between days and nights, though he was home every day. My own schedule remained two day shifts, two night shifts, followed by four days off. Our son was now attending school, and childcare was challenging at times, but my mother generously stepped in whenever we needed her, without hesitation. Between the three of us—my husband, myself, and my mother—we managed to make it work.

Personally, I was merely existing, going through the motions day in and day out. At work, crew members rotated annually, and I often found myself working with people I didn't particularly want to spend my time with. It was the luck of the draw and not all personalities meshed well. Unfortunately, on one particular shift I found myself clashing with too many colleagues.

I had no choice in the matter and was stuck with some of these guys for three years. It was far from ideal, but I found ways to cope by minimizing contact with them while at work. During our downtime, I would remove myself, keeping busy while they all hung out together.

One day, as I was sitting in the fire prevention office working on a course, I noticed one of the guys come downstairs and quickly pass by the office. I didn't pay much attention, as I honestly didn't care what he was up to. A short time later he reappeared, this time carrying bags of takeout food. I watched as he sauntered past my open office door and headed back upstairs. I sat there for a moment as the reality sank in; they had ordered food and didn't even bother to include me.

Feeling a mix of curiosity and dread, I got up from behind the desk and made my way upstairs. I was a sucker for punishment and needed to see it with my own eyes. As I reached the day room, there they were, three of them sitting at the table eating. It was exactly as I had thought. They had done a group food order and completely excluded me. My heart sank a little but only for a second. It quickly turned into a deep, gutted anger. Shaking my head, I made my way back downstairs to the quiet solitude of the office, feeling more isolated than ever.

This incident was the first of many and a reminder of the underlying tension and lack of camaraderie that plagued my shift. It wasn't just the exclusion from a meal; it was the persistent feeling of being an outsider in what was supposed to be a brotherhood. I resolved to focus on my work and keep my distance, knowing that in time, there would be change again. But until then, I would have to find strength in my solitude and remain professional despite the personal slights.

I had been diligently working on my personal growth for a while and decided it was time to reward myself with a solo tropical vacation. I spent a week in Cancun, Mexico, embarking on a glorious adventure of self-discovery. During my trip, I chose not to make friends or engage in conversations beyond the necessary interactions with the waitstaff. My goal was to embrace solitude and avoid distractions. It turned out to be the best gift I could have given myself. The week away taught me invaluable lessons about self-reliance and inner peace.

While traveling abroad, my phone remained in airplane mode, allowing me to fully disconnect. However, when I landed back on Canadian soil and switched my phone back on, I was bombarded with a torrent of text notifications from a group chat. I quickly realized that it was a thread involving all union members. Hundreds of messages had accumulated during my absence, making it impossible to catch up by scrolling through them. Puzzled and concerned, I immediately called my union president.

"What the fuck is going on?" I asked, perplexed. "I just landed and got all these group texts."

"I'll make a long story short," he replied. "The chief was fired. No warning, no explanations."

I was stunned. My mind raced, trying to process this sudden and shocking news. What the fuck? Why? I had so many questions and so few answers. Upon arriving home, I met with a few of my colleagues to gather updates on the situation. Unfortunately, no one had concrete information, and our employers maintained an unsettling silence. This radio silence persisted for a year, leaving us in a state of constant uncertainty.

During this time a temporary deputy chief was brought in to help us regain some semblance of normalcy. As firefighters, we knew our jobs and performed them well, even without a clear leader. I took great pride in how we banded together and continued to serve our community with dedication and professionalism, while behind closed doors was complete chaos.

Then, another bombshell dropped. We were informed that two of our firefighters would be moving into chief positions. Initially, I felt a surge of excitement. This was the first time anyone had moved internally from the floor into a management role—a significant milestone in our department's history. Traditionally in the fire service, firefighters progressed through the ranks from firefighter to captain, and eventually into deputy chief and fire chief positions before retirement. This internal promotion structure was supposed to foster healthy career progression and boost morale.

I believed having our own firefighters transition into chief roles would be advantageous, as they were already familiar with the department's inner workings and had personal connections with all of us. However, I couldn't have been more wrong. It quickly became evident that there had been widespread corruption behind the scenes. These promotions had been part of a larger, sinister plan. Instead of celebration, we were being faced with a period of turmoil and disillusionment.

The situation created a massive conflict of interest, intertwining the union and the new boss. The atmosphere buzzed with tension and speculation around the matter, with no solution in sight. My trust and confidence in the leadership for both the union and the department eroded completely. It was an extremely unsettling feeling, leaving me deeply concerned about the well-being of my colleagues and myself. We were navigating uncharted waters and only time would tell as the path ahead was fraught with uncertainty and distrust.

CHAPTER 23

Never Off Duty

Not only did I have the honor of impacting lives while on duty, but I also had the privilege to do so off duty. January 31, 2021, stands out as a day that profoundly affected many lives, including my own. My family and I were leaving early in the morning for a day of skiing in the mountains. As usual, we were running late because of me. We finally got everything loaded into the truck and pulled out of the garage. I immediately noticed heavy smoke in the air, even though it was still dark. Something felt off. We pulled out of the driveway and onto the street.

"There's a structure fire somewhere," I said to my family.

I instinctively knew it. I was sitting forward and alert in my seat, and my eyes were quickly scanning the surroundings, trying to locate the source of the smoke. My husband was driving slowly and looking intently along the way. As we drove around the bend to the next street over, the smoke grew thicker. I knew we were close, but I still couldn't pinpoint where it was coming from. We were creeping along the street, laser-focused on finding the fire and having some back-and-forth discussion. We got about halfway up the street and were able to narrow it down to two houses. We pulled into the driveway of one and my husband began honking the horn to draw attention or wake people up. We both jumped out of the truck and started running in different directions, trying to locate the source of the fire. The smoke was billowing and extremely thick, making it hard to breathe. Processing the urgency of the situation, I grabbed my phone out of my pocket and called the firehall directly. Visibility was getting worse, and my eyes and throat were burning, so I ran around the leeward side of the house to avoid some of the smoke.

"Fire emergency for what area?" My colleague calmly answered the phone.

I quickly told him it was me and that there was a structure fire. Even though I wasn't certain which house it was, I knew I needed to alert the crew and get the fire truck rolling in this direction. I scoured the front of the house I was standing at for house numbers, but the front was still under construction and had none.

"It's this one!" I heard my husband holler from around back.

I didn't have an address, so I started looking around, trying to provide possible landmarks for reference. Realizing this wasn't helping and I needed an actual address, I sprinted to the house next door. I noted their house number and relayed that the fire was in the house beside it. My colleague took the information slowly and then calmly asked me for my name and phone number. Frustration surged through me; I had already identified myself at the beginning of the call and assumed he knew by now.

"It's fucking Lynnette!" I hollered aggressively.

I hung up the phone and sprinted to the front door. Making a fist, I hammered on the door as hard as I could. I cupped my hands and peered through the glass, but the house was completely dark inside. It was early in the morning, and I assumed everyone was still asleep. Just then, my husband came running up beside me, breathless and with a sense of urgency.

"The whole back of the house is on fire!" His eyes were wide with terror.

I started pounding on the door again. The gravity of the situation hit even harder, and I knew we needed to get inside right away!

I stopped for a second to tell my husband that we needed to kick the door in when suddenly a light flicked on, catching both of our attention. Standing at the top of the stairs was a very pregnant woman, flanked by two little girls. They looked terrified!

"Your house is on fire! Open the door!" I screamed while frantically pointing toward the lock.

I think it took a moment for my words to register. Wide-eyed and with a visible mix of fear and confusion, the woman made her way down the stairs and unlocked the door. As soon as it swung open, both my husband and I urgently repeated that the house was on fire and they needed to get out!

I noted the two small girls with her and quickly asked if there was anyone else in the house. I thought I heard her say there was one more, so I took off running, bolting up two sets of stairs to the top floor. I scanned the bedroom quickly but saw no one. I raced down one set of stairs to the main floor and ran down the hallway, scanning every room to the end. Nothing. I hurried back to the entry landing and asked her again if there was anyone else in the house. She confirmed that it was just the three of them and a surge of relief washed over me. We asked her where their coats and boots were, and she pointed to the entry closet. My husband and I quickly started going through the closet, pulling out coats and boots. We asked each of the girls' which items were theirs. We were both crouched down in front of the girls, reassuring them that they were safe, and everything was going to be okay as we got them dressed. Out of nowhere, a man appeared at the front door. My husband and he knew each other. He was a neighbor who had seen our truck parked in the driveway with its doors open and left running and he stopped to help. The little girls were both dressed warmly now, so we guided them to go with him. He took them outside to his warm truck for safety.

Now my attention shifted entirely to helping the woman get her coat and boots from the closet. She was talking on her phone while I struggled to get her boots onto her feet. Once that task was complete, I stood up and turned back to the closet to fetch her coat. As I asked her which one she wanted, she suddenly dashed up the stairs to the main floor and headed straight for the pantry. Alarmed, I chased after her, asking what she was doing and reminding her that we needed to go! I was extremely confused, trying to understand why she was ignoring the urgency of the situation. When I finally caught up to her, she was rummaging through the bottom of the pantry. My first thought was that she was looking for her purse or something valuable or important. She was still talking on her phone, but I interrupted.

"What are you doing?" I asked again so I could help her find whatever it was.

"I'm looking for a fire extinguisher," she hurriedly explained.

I heard what she said but at that precise moment something unusual caught my eye. I glanced away from her as my gaze was drawn to the wall beside the pantry. Time seemed to freeze as I focused on the glow of orange through the seam in the wall. I tracked the glow upward to the ceiling. To my horror, I saw flames racing across the entire ceiling behind the recessed lighting. I mentally noted in that moment that there wasn't a single wisp of smoke in the house. I also noted the complete silence as none of the smoke detectors were going off.

I snapped back to reality, grabbed both of her hands firmly, and locked eyes.

"That's not going to work. *We have to go!*" I said sternly.

Thankfully, she understood my urgency in that moment, and we abandoned the pantry and hurried back downstairs. I helped her put on her coat, then opened the door to the garage where her car was parked. I closed the door behind us and pushed the button to open the garage bay door, then assisted her into her vehicle. As she settled into the driver's seat, I looked up and my eyes met my husband's. He was back in his truck with our son, and I motioned for him to move out of the way. He nodded in understanding and began backing out of the driveway to make room for her to pull out. She drove her car out of the garage and onto the street. As she pulled away, I followed her out of the garage, and my attention was immediately drawn to the sound of a siren and the flashing lights of an approaching fire truck.

I ran down the driveway and onto the street to meet the fire truck. As soon as it pulled up to the curb, I went straight to the captain and informed him that everyone was safely out of the house. After relaying all the critical information I knew he needed, I jumped in to help pull the hose off the truck and straighten it for water so the firefighters could quickly get water flowing to tackle the blaze. Once the hoses were in place, I took a moment to step back and survey the scene. From this vantage point, I could see the flames lighting up the night sky and devouring the back of the house. A hose line was extended to the front door, and firefighters were positioned, ready to make their entry. I watched as they opened the door and directed a powerful stream of water inside. As the water hit, the ceiling collapsed with a thunderous crash. I stood there, frozen in shock. Just mere moments earlier, we had been standing in that very spot that was now reduced to a pile of smoking debris. The reality of how close we had come to disaster hit me hard and left me momentarily paralyzed.

I snapped back into action and scanned the area for my husband's truck. I spotted it parked a short distance away, so I sprinted over and climbed into the passenger seat. I urgently told him that I needed him to drive me home because I had to get my car and head to the firehall to get my gear. The fire had escalated to an "all call," which meant it required all available members to respond. I was no longer going on a planned ski trip to the mountains; I was going to work. In less than a minute, we arrived back at our house. I kissed my family and told them I would see them later. I dashed inside and up the stairs to quickly change out of my ski fleece and into suitable work attire. I raced through the house, grabbing my keys and a few essentials, then got in my car and pulled it out of the garage. As I sped toward the firehall, I had to pull over several times as more fire trucks passed in the opposite direction, racing toward the fire. When I arrived at the firehall, I sprinted inside and swiftly donned my gear. I had arrived at the same time as a few other firefighters, so we rallied together and quickly hopped into a truck, with me behind the wheel, and headed back to the scene. Once there, I immediately located command, handed in my accountability tags, received my task assignment, and got to work. It was just like any other fire operation, except I had already been up close and personal with this one, so I knew what the scene would be like.

Sometime later, I noticed that my husband and son had backed into a driveway across the street from the fire and were watching the entire scene unfold. This was the first time they had ever seen me in action. Over the years, they had heard countless stories about the various fires I had battled and the things I did on the job, but they had never witnessed it firsthand. I was immediately filled with immense pride. I was deeply dedicated to the work I did and having them see me perform my duties felt incredibly rewarding. I walked over to the truck to check in with them, and my son immediately wrapped his arms around me in a big hug. His eyes were wide with excitement as he recounted details of what he had seen me do. Then he started firing off a barrage of questions about everything else that was going on. I answered his questions with a smile and felt a sense of honor and accomplishment, not just in my work, but in the fact that my family could see it too. After a few minutes, I told them that I had to get back to work and gave them each a hug and a kiss. They returned to watching the scene as I went back to my position on a hose line.

A little while later, I was standing in the middle of the street in the rehabilitation area with a few of my colleagues. We had taken our air packs off and were in rest and recovery to cool down and hydrate. Suddenly I had the distinct feeling that someone else was watching me. I turned slowly and saw a man walking up the street toward me with determined purpose. He was laser-focused on me. As he drew closer, I noticed the serious expression on his face.

"I understand you're the one who saved my family this morning," he said.

"Yes, I did," I confirmed.

His face softened immediately, and without hesitation, he pulled me into the biggest hug. We stood there and embraced for a moment as he repeatedly thanked me. Tears welled up in my eyes and I fought to hold back my emotions. His gratitude touched me deeply. We talked for a couple of minutes and then parted ways.

I hadn't fully processed what had happened that morning. The moment we got the family out of the house, I had switched into work mode and was focused entirely on the task at hand. I had been on the scene for quite a while now, fully immersed in my duties, with no time to reflect on everything until that man approached me and thanked me. Everything had unfolded so rapidly that I hadn't even comprehended the magnitude of our actions. We had saved that man's family.

Once everything was under control, we assisted the homeowner in salvaging a great number of valuables from the garage. The fire was extinguished so we cleaned up and cleared from the scene to return to the firehall. Once there, we began the process of cleaning all the equipment and restocking the trucks to get them back in service. As we worked, a few of my colleagues approached me with questions about what had happened. Some had heard that I was the one who had initially called in the fire; others were unaware of my involvement. Amidst all the hustle and bustle, I still hadn't fully processed the events of the morning yet. Adrenaline was now surging through my veins again as I recounted the story to them. As I narrated the details, I noticed that that my hands were trembling. The realization hit me just then that I was more shaken up than I had initially thought. Replaying the events brought back the intensity of the crisis and I felt the weight of the experience settling in.

My colleagues congratulated me with handshakes, high fives, and the odd pat on the back. Their smiles and words of encouragement affirmed that I had done a good job. I could see genuine pride in some of their eyes, and it felt incredibly rewarding. I knew how much their recognition meant. But it wasn't just about the praise; it was about being part of a team that truly valued and acknowledged my contributions.

My husband and I were riding an incredible high for a few days. We couldn't stop talking about what had transpired and the roles that we played. It still seemed surreal how everything had unfolded. The timing felt almost divine and whatever force had orchestrated it was extraordinarily powerful. We had been exactly where we needed to be, precisely when we needed to be there. Naturally, we found ourselves playing out various "what if" scenarios and imagining different outcomes. But we quickly shut those thoughts down and reminded each other that the situation had resulted in the absolute best possible outcome for everyone involved. We both felt a deep sense of gratitude and awe at how everything had aligned so perfectly.

I waited patiently for the family to share their experience on social media, respecting that it was their story to tell first. Once they did, I reached out and asked for their permission to share my perspective of the event. They graciously agreed. When I posted my account of the story, it quickly went viral. People were shocked by the details I revealed, as many had no idea about the dramatic events that had occurred that day.

A couple of days later, I received word that my boss had finally conducted a briefing with the media. I was anxious to see the coverage. I sat and wondered if my efforts and accomplishment had been enough to be acknowledged. Would saving a family from a burning house finally be enough to prove myself? Over the years, I had grown accustomed to seeking their approval and constantly striving to prove my worth.

While I was scrolling through Facebook, a picture of the house fire on the city's page suddenly appeared on my feed. My heart skipped a beat as I paused and then leaned in to read the caption.

"As many of you have heard, the Dawson Creek Fire Department attended a house fire in the 900 block of 89 Avenue over the weekend. The crew

responded with 4 apparatus and 21 firefighters. On arrival, the roof was fully involved with extension into the living area. The fire was contained to the residence top floor and roof, and those that were inside are safe. Looking for tips on everyday fire safety and prevention? Visit the city website."

I sat there completely motionless; every part of my body was stiff with tension. Emotions churned inside me as a storm of unsettling feelings and questioning thoughts were darting through my mind. Was that really all they had to say about the whole event? Seriously? I was in disbelief. But in all honesty, I was not entirely surprised. I was hurt, but that hurt quickly transformed into anger over the fact that my actions had been so easily dismissed. I couldn't help but shake my head at their ignorance. I had been hopeful for applause, but I suppose stunned silence was equally appropriate. I put myself aside and all I could imagine was how incredible it would have made them all look if they had managed to get past their egos and used the headlines and story as an opportunity to promote the department. I envisioned something like, "Off-duty firefighter saves family from house fire. This is the caliber of firefighters we have in this department that your tax dollars are paying for. They use their professionalism, training and skills even while off duty to keep your community safe." This narrative would have been especially powerful since we had been constantly told by this man prior to him becoming a boss that the public didn't like us and thought we didn't work very hard for what we got paid. I was convinced this would've been the perfect way to show the public otherwise and to demonstrate our dedication and heroism. But it seemed I was alone in my thinking.

It wasn't just about not promoting the department; deep down, I knew the reason was because it was me. I could safely assume that if anyone else in the department had performed the same heroic act, they would've received credit, acknowledgment, and probably even an award or medal for their actions. Instead, I was met with silence and disregard. The reaction from friends, family, and members of the community was swift and clear as I received a flood of unprompted phone calls and messages from them expressing their disgust at the media release. Their outrage mirrored my own feelings, and it was a small comfort to know that others recognized the injustice. I didn't need to respond with any grand statements, explanations, or even give any names. In fact, I didn't need to say anything at all. People had now seen it with their own eyes, and they knew exactly who was behind it.

When the chaos settled a few weeks later, we had the pleasure of meeting with the couple from the fire. They arrived at our home bearing gifts of appreciation and gratitude, which were a touching gesture that spoke volumes about their thankfulness. We sat down together at the dining room table and engaged in a captivating conversation. As we talked, we each shared our perspectives on the fire and recounted our experiences and emotions from that morning. It was incredible to hear their sides of the story. She was at home alone with the girls—snuggling upstairs in bed with one, while the other slept in her room down on the main floor—and he was already at work when he got the frantic call from her. Recounting the immense relief they each felt once he arrived on the scene and their family unit was safe once again. Their heartfelt appreciation for our actions was my medal of honor. In turn, my husband and I shared our own accounts. I explained how my instincts and training had driven me to act and how everything had unfolded from my perspective.

Then my husband shared how he had followed my lead, and then what he witnessed from the back of the house that no one else had. We each shared how we had felt in those intense moments. This exchange was more than just a conversation. It gave us all the opportunity to connect on a deeper level and fill in so many questionable blanks about the event. We had pieced together a comprehensive narrative and were able to understand all the different facets of that morning.

We were in the middle of our conversation when our son walked up and presented the couple with drawings he had made of their house on fire. At first, I was horrified and tried to stop him, as I feared it would be a painful reminder and entirely inappropriate. But the woman graciously intervened and assured me it was okay. She accepted the drawings with a warm smile and invited our son to explain his artwork. I watched as he eagerly pointed out each detail in his pictures and carefully described the flames, the house, and the rescue. As he spoke, my initial horror gave way to a swelling sense of pride and understanding. It dawned on me that his drawings were his way of processing what he had witnessed and felt. Until that moment, I hadn't fully grasped the depth of his experience, assuming he had been shielded from the worst of it since he stayed in the truck the entire time. But now I realized he had his own unique perspective on the event, and this was his way of telling his story. I was immensely proud of his bravery and insight and horribly disappointed in myself for how I had been consumed with my own perspective and hadn't considered his. After that moment, my husband and I encouraged him to share his thoughts and feelings with us whenever he needed to. It became clear that we all had our own work to do, as we were each processing the impact of that house fire in our own ways. Truth be told, the experience changed us all.

CHAPTER 24

A Hero And An Angel

The house fire story and its impact didn't end there. A couple of months after the fire, I received a heartwarming message on Facebook from the pregnant woman we had rescued. Her words were joyous as she shared the news that their newest family member had arrived. They had welcomed a beautiful, healthy baby boy into the world.

I was filled with happiness as I read all the details she shared about their son's birth and admired the sweet picture she had attached. As I continued reading, I gasped when I reached the part where she shared his full name. She explained that his name contained the initials L. W., chosen in honor of us, their angels: Lynnette and Wade. Tears welled up in my eyes and my breath escaped me. I reread the words several times just to make sure I was understanding them correctly. I sat there for a few moments, trying to catch my breath as tears streamed freely down my face. It was the most precious gesture I had ever received. My husband walked into the room and was instantly concerned when he saw me crying.

"Sit down. There's something I need to tell you," I said.

The expression on his face made me realize too late that my words had made him think something terrible had happened. I quickly corrected and ensured him that it was a good thing.

"The couple from the house fire had their baby," I explained.

Relief washed over his face as he took the seat next to me. I handed him my phone so he could read the message himself. I knew I would never be able to keep my composure long enough to say the words out loud. He began reading with a smile, but I could tell when he reached the part about the baby's name as his expression shifted to one of shock and deep emotion. He slowly raised his tear-filled eyes and looked at me. Just like me, he was trying to process what he had just read.

"Holy fuck," he said in a shaky whisper.

We stood and embraced each other, allowing the flood of emotions to surface. In that moment neither of us needed to speak; we fully understood the magnitude of the honor we had just received.

I honestly didn't know how to process it all. My job had always been professional and impersonal, and I had learned to dissociate myself from the emotional weight of the work that I did. But this situation was different, and I couldn't do that because it had become profoundly personal. These incredible people were mere acquaintances before the fire and now their newborn child bore our initials in his name as a permanent reminder of our connection. It was overwhelming.

I had been called a hero and now an angel. The word *hero* had always been extremely difficult for me to absorb, and *angel* even more so. To me, I simply did what needed to be done that day. What I was trained to do. There was no hesitation or second-guessing, and my husband had acted just as instinctively. I knew in my heart that our acts were heroic and with a little time I was able to fully accept it. We had literally saved four lives! It was the ultimate personal achievement and the pinnacle of my career. The magnitude of our actions hit me hard, especially knowing that as a result, their child now carried our legacy in his name. This act had transformed what I considered a professional deed into a deeply personal one and created a lasting connection with a family we had once only distantly known. The fact that they wanted to honor us through their child was both humbling and significant. It had become a story that would be told for generations. Our son and their children now shared a bond that had been forged in the heat of crisis, one they would be able to recount together throughout their lives. I hope that as they grow up, they become friends and share our extraordinary tale of heroism.

I achieved something unprecedented and reaped *the* greatest reward from it. I had received the highest form of acknowledgment and recognition. Through this experience, I had finally reached a level of self-acceptance and understanding where I no longer needed validation from my bosses or departmental accolades. The recognition I had received from that family and, more significantly, from myself was enough.

I was still struggling to process the complex emotions that were tied to the experience months later. I often found myself in tears and feeling extremely emotional. These tears weren't out of sadness. They were a release of overwhelming feelings that I was unable to immediately comprehend, and it took me a while to understand this emotional catharsis. To navigate these emotions, I did a lot of journaling to pour my thoughts and feelings onto paper. Additionally, I engaged in talk therapy with my counselor multiple times. These methods were what allowed me to be honest with myself and recognize that this aspect of my job had become deeply personal. Even though I was off duty when the event occurred, my identity as a firefighter and being committed to keeping my community safe had remained central to who I was. I had diligently established healthy coping mechanisms to detach myself from the traumatic experiences I encountered on the job, helping to reinforce that these events weren't personal.

However, this particular experience defied that separation. It took time for me to reconcile that I could embody both the roles as the professional firefighter and the emotional human being. I learned that it was okay for me to integrate these identities. I didn't have to be two separate entities like I had taught myself to become. I could, in fact, be a whole person, a human, and a firefighter simultaneously.

CHAPTER 25

You're Not Going To Cry

While processing my reaction to the house fire and working through the varied emotions, some long-suppressed memories resurfaced. I vividly recalled a conversation I had in the dayroom with a captain and a relatively new firefighter shortly before I was hired.

"What are you going to do when you see a dead body?' the captain asked.

"I don't know because I've never seen one," I jokingly replied.

The captain then turned very serious.

"I'll tell you what you're not going to do," he said emphatically. "You're not going to cry."

His words echoed ones I'd heard as a child. Much like before, I nodded as if I understood his reasoning, but realistically, I didn't. I then took the opportunity to redirect and asked the other firefighter if he had ever seen a dead body, to which he replied that he hadn't. I followed with the same question that had been asked to me.

"What are you going to do when you see one?" I asked curiously.

He admitted that he didn't know how he would react, but he was confident that he could handle it. The captain reassured him and affirmed his confidence. Our conversation then turned to the topic of dealing with a deceased child. I mentioned that I didn't have any children, so I wasn't sure how I would react. The other firefighter had recently become a father and expressed uncertainty about how such an event would affect him. Even though we had the same response, I noticed a significant difference. He didn't receive the same directive about what his emotional reaction was *allowed* to be. I absorbed the captain's statement to me, telling me not to cry and unknowingly allowed it to shape my behavior and emotional responses going forward.

For many years I witnessed extremely traumatic events and worked some terribly disturbing calls that could have, or should have, stirred up an emotional response such as crying—but I didn't. I could vividly recall having my hands wrapped around the tiny chest of a lifeless two-week-old infant, desperately performing chest compressions in the effort to revive her. Unfortunately, the outcome wasn't successful, and I felt utter devastation. But I was emotionally armored and held back any tears or feelings of grief because to me, crying over the job equaled weakness, and I was determined not to be perceived as weak. Instead, I channeled my emotions into anger, as that seemed more socially and culturally acceptable. I often found myself becoming intensely angry over minor things that didn't warrant such a reaction. At home, this anger manifested in destructive ways, and I would punch holes in walls, throw things, and yell. These outbursts became my outlet of being able to release the pent-up emotions I refused to express through tears.

Over the years, I had become a very angry person. Anger became my default response in any given situation, even those that could have been easily resolved with simple communication. Instead of calmly addressing issues, I would become intensely angry and defensive, which only exacerbated the problem. As I began to unravel my emotions, I discovered that anger was a common response to events that seemed unfair, situations where I felt betrayed by others, or instances where I had ever been made a victim. I vehemently rejected the idea of being a victim though. The word itself was repulsive to me; there was no fucking way I was one. In my mind, I was too strong to ever be a victim, and I refused to accept such a label. I was determined to find another explanation, so I delved deep into self-reflection and brutally honest introspection. Much to my dismay, I realized that I had indeed been a victim. The anger I had been using as a shield was a cover-up for the genuine pain and injustice I had endured over the years.

Acknowledging this truth was a pivotal moment for me. I had to confront the reality that my anger was not just a misguided emotion but an honest response to my experiences. I recognized that there was such a thing as healthy anger, which was a constructive and justified reaction to being wronged. However, the anger I had been displaying was far from healthy. It was a destructive force that masked my true feelings and prevented me from healing. Understanding that my anger was a normal reaction did provide some comfort, but it was still difficult for me to fully accept. Admitting that I had been a victim required a level of vulnerability I wasn't accustomed to.

The more aware I became, the more I could see things for what they really were. Taking off the blinders allowed me to gain a much clearer understanding of myself. A phrase kept showing up in my awareness: "Your body keeps the score. What you don't express, your body will suppress." This concept intrigued me. I had always understood that emotions are meant to be expressed, as that is their natural purpose. However, I didn't understand that substituting the correct emotion with what seemed more suitable in that moment was unhealthy. My mind was blown when I learned that suppressing my true emotions didn't mean they simply disappeared. Instead, they attached themselves to my tissues and my organs, which contributed to physical and emotional "dis-ease." This insight was eye-opening and helped me understand what was happening with my own body. Suppressing my emotions wasn't just a mental issue; it was a physiological one too.

Suppressing my urge to cry and bottling up that emotion resulted in a persistent tightness in my chest and the near-constant feeling of being short of breath. Even though I was active and in great physical shape, I often felt winded on scene. I had always attributed this to nerves or anxiety and convinced myself that it was just part of who I was. I had suffered with that silent companion throughout my career. Imagine my surprise when I began to allow myself to process and genuinely feel my emotions. It was as if a heavy weight had been lifted off my chest, and suddenly, I could breathe easier. The simple act of crying to bring me such an immense physical relief left me dumbfounded. I had been carrying around a tremendous amount of suppressed emotional baggage that needed an outlet. For years, the only release I had allowed myself was through rigorous exercise at the gym or, regrettably, through angry outbursts like putting my fist into a wall.

It was overwhelming to fully grasp at first; eventually though, it made perfect sense. Being honest with myself showed me that just because I had managed to carry a heavy burden didn't mean it wasn't insanely fucking heavy. The weight had been wreaking havoc on my body and now that I understood the true extent of what I had been enduring, everything became clear.

When I had surrendered to the tears after the house fire, I realized that was the reason why they didn't stop flowing for quite some time. As I mentioned before, I wasn't sad. It turned out that the tears were purely a healthy release—and a much needed one at that! As the weight of my emotions lifted, I felt unrestrained and much lighter. Giving myself permission to cry was one of the greatest gifts I could have given to myself and my family. They never deserved the angry version of me, and it was painful to know that's who I had become just to survive.

CHAPTER 26

I Used To Be Fun

I had been functioning in a trauma response without even knowing it for over a decade. My career and my experiences had become so intertwined with my identity that I had succumbed to the belief that I would always be like this. I convinced myself that my experiences had hardened me and served as proof that I was strong and capable of handling anything life threw at me. But in reality, I could not have been more wrong!

I had turned my experiences into a place of residence rather than a place of reference. Instead of learning from them and moving forward, I had built my entire life around my past traumas. I had completely armored up and constructed emotional barriers so impenetrable that I existed fully immersed in my trauma. The weight of my past dictated every aspect of my present, clouded my vision, and stifled my growth. Each day felt like a relentless battle just to maintain my hardened exterior. In this fortified state, I wasn't truly living, and I sure as hell wasn't thriving. I was merely existing.

I lived my life in constant fear and was always envisioning the worst-case scenario in my mind. I had convinced myself that by anticipating every possible threat, I could stay ahead and keep myself safe. I was either trapped in the past, or I was fixated on the future, and neither of those allowed me to fully experience the present moment. This relentless fear transformed me into an absolute control freak, and I wore that title like it was a badge of honor. I micromanaged everyone and everything that was close to me because I believed that if I could control the small details, then I would have some semblance of control in my life. My mind was always on high alert, and I took worrying to an extreme level that I hadn't even thought was possible. I scanned my environment constantly, in search of potential threats, and prepared for danger at every turn. This hypervigilance gave me a false sense of security and safety, making me believe I could never be caught off guard because I was always two steps ahead of any harm. However, this illusion of control came at a significant cost. By trying to foresee and manage every possible danger, I disconnected myself from the present and missed out on joy and precious moments.

I used to be fun!

That realization hit me one day like a tidal wave. Somewhere along the way, I had become so fucking serious about everything all the time that I literally didn't know how to have fun anymore. I remembered what fun looked like and for a few moments I basked in the memories of how I used to be. I was easy-going, always social, and out all the time with friends. I had a lot of friends, and I was known for my sarcasm and sense of humor. Oh man, how I loved to laugh! And dancing was my ultimate joy. There was nothing I loved more than dancing the night away with friends. I knew how to have fun. As I reminisced, I wondered when all that had changed. It wasn't a sudden shift because that would've been noticeable. It must have been a slow, gradual erosion of my carefree spirit that was imperceptible at the time, but completely undeniable now. I tried to pinpoint the moment it all faded away, but it eluded me.

I felt a deep sadness when I realized that I didn't have many friends left. Over time, my circle had dwindled to just a few people that I could truly trust and allow close to me. The numerous betrayals and deep hurts that I had experienced had left scars so deep that I found it easier and less painful to keep others at a safe distance. I built emotional walls and convinced myself that solitude was a safer alternative because inside those walls I could control the threat of potential pain or hurt.

I refused to ask for help, and when I did receive it, it rarely met my standards anyway, which made it seem easier to just do everything myself. I became a workaholic and constantly immersed myself in projects to keep busy. I was running on empty, yet I couldn't make myself rest or relax. Any type of decision-making filled me with dread because I was fearful of making the wrong choices. Over time, I had become a people pleaser with invisible boundaries, yet I always wondered why they were continually being violated. I prioritized everyone else's needs over my own and allowed people to walk all over me to avoid conflict. My trust issues were extreme. I didn't trust myself, let alone anyone else. This lack of trust encouraged my need for external validation and placed my self-worth entirely on the opinions of others. This cycle of self-imposed isolation and overwork left me exhausted and disconnected from my true self.

From the beginning of my career, I had established bulletproof coping mechanisms to handle the traumatic calls I responded to and the horrific things I witnessed and dealt with in my job. I knew these strategies were essential for my mental and emotional well-being. I had a trusted counselor with whom I had built a strong, supportive connection. This therapeutic relationship was important because it provided me with a safe space to process my experiences and emotions. I journaled faithfully in grave detail so

I could capture the facts to prevent my mind from creating false narratives that could amplify my stress and anxiety. Writing everything down served as a powerful tool for me to self-reflect and maintain mental clarity. Exercise was another cornerstone of my coping strategy. I had always been committed to a rigorous workout routine, so I used that physical release to my advantage for the tension and stress that could accumulate from my job. These coping mechanisms were nonnegotiable from day one. They were pillars of my routine, designed to safeguard my well-being amidst the chaos and trauma of my work. These practices served me well and provided me the stability and resilience I needed whenever I was faced with challenges.

On the flip side, I had never considered that I would need strategies in place for coping with being personally attacked. Unfortunately, instead of leaning into my healthy coping mechanisms, I developed unhealthy ones that were distractions. I kept myself insanely busy maintaining a never-ending to-do list. If I wasn't working, I was painting the house, or renovating, or tackling projects in the yard. I became a workaholic, always on the go. I accepted every overtime shift and covered for colleagues whenever they needed. I simply could not sit still. This constant busyness had given me a false sense of being productive and successful. But in all honesty, I was neither productive nor successful. I was trying to outrun myself so I didn't have to acknowledge or feel the truth. The plethora of activities were a desperate attempt to escape myself, but they weren't working. No matter where I went, there I was. It was really fucking annoying running into myself everywhere I went. I found that the busier I kept myself, the less time I had to feel, and the less I had to outrun my shadow. However, the only thing this frantic pace did was busy me straight into a burnout. I was miserable, exhausted, fearful, and filled with shame. My avoidance strategies had backfired.

The truth was, I had to turn around and face myself. I had to stop running and own my role in my own suffering. I had hidden the truth and kept secrets for so long that the anger I felt inevitably turned inward. Instead of hating the men that hurt me, I hated myself. I couldn't force them to accept me, to see me, or to treat me the way I deserved to be treated. No matter how much value I brought to the table, I couldn't make my colleagues, or my bosses see it when they chose not to.

On the flip side, certain men at the department had repeatedly shown me who they were, but I had refused to believe the truth. I ignored their actions because I didn't want to see the reality. Their behavior was the greatest form of communication, and I had accepted their behaviors and mistreatment as "normal." My self-worth had eroded to such a low point that being disrespected and mistreated became the routine I expected. It had become their normal, too, because they had gotten away with it for so fucking long that it became their default way of treating me. What I had tolerated, continued. Lies, deception, backstabbing, manipulation, discrimination, and bullying; I had allowed these to persist because I refused to accept the truth of who they were. I had to let go of the idealized version of who they could be and accept the reality of who they had shown themselves to be.

Over the years, I had caught these men in countless lies. Each time I dared to speak up and expose the truth, I was immediately gaslit. They would turn the situation around and insist that I was making everything about myself and taking things way too personally. Instead of owning their dishonesty, they would flip the script and blame me for the fires they started and the chaos they created. They masterfully convinced me that the real issue wasn't their mistreatment of me; rather, it was my reaction to it. In the end, I carried an immense amount of shame for allowing things to go as far as they did. Their manipulation pushed me to believe that I didn't deserve any better and trapped me in a cycle of self-doubt and unworthiness.

When I finally allowed myself to see the truth, it shattered my heart to know that I had completely sacrificed my authenticity for acceptance. In my desperate attempt to fit in, I had judged myself through their eyes and shape-shifted to become who I thought they wanted me to be. Everything about me had changed and it troubled me deeply that I couldn't pinpoint exactly when it all happened. Had the complete dismantling of myself been a gradual transformation over time, or a continuation of the shifts I had to make in the beginning, dependent on who I was working with? This was a question I was unable to solidly answer. However, what I did know for sure was that this was never what I had wanted. All I ever truly desired was to belong. To have that feeling of acceptance, to feel safe and secure, and to be valued for who I genuinely was. Instead, I found myself drowning in the compromise of my authenticity. I was so deeply immersed in this false identity that I couldn't even see the possibility of rising to the surface.

As I stood in front of the mirror, my fingers naturally navigating the last button on my uniform shirt, I couldn't help but feel a profound disconnect with the reflection staring back at me. My eyes slowly studied the empty shell of a woman that once was vibrant and spirited in that uniform. In her place stood a hollow shell, consumed by darkness and pain. With each meticulous adjustment, a wave of self-loathing washed over me, not directed at the job or my colleagues, but at the person I had become. The uniform that was once a symbol of pride and purpose now felt like a facade, a flimsy cover-up for the lies, pain, and secrets festering within me. Yet no amount of fabric could conceal the truth from my own gaze. Deep down, I knew the source of my turmoil, the reasons for the darkness and secrets that plagued me.

In that moment of brutal self-reflection, I despised the woman staring back at me. She was everything I never wanted to be. A betrayal of my beliefs, my morals, my values, and my standards. How the fuck had I allowed myself to stray so far from the path that I once tread with conviction? Every glance in the mirror was a painful reminder of the ways in which I had abandoned myself, betrayed my own standards, and turned a blind eye to the glaring truths that confronted me time and time again.

The bitterness I felt toward myself was exemplified when I acknowledged the relationships I had fractured in my journey of self-destruction. Those I loved had become unwitting casualties of my refusal to confront the harsh realities of my actions. In my desperation to evade accountability, I had turned the people I loved into the enemy because I didn't want to face what I had done to them. That included me. I was also the enemy.

In reaction to my surroundings, I had morphed into someone unrecognizable, straying far from my true essence. Instead of nurturing my authentic self, I had erected walls of defense. As a result, my confidence waned, my self-esteem plummeted, and my self-doubt consumed me. I was adrift, unfamiliar with the person staring back at me in the mirror. Yet at the same time I despised the stranger I had become. I was lost and shattered but felt the faintest hint of longing to rediscover my identity.

CHAPTER 27

I Am a Legend

Now that I had faced the truth about myself, it was time to get really fucking honest with every part of my being. I needed to do the one thing I had consistently refused to do all along; I had to get vulnerable. *Cringe!* It was the most crucial and necessary step so that I could heal. While I had been diligently avoiding vulnerability and shielding myself from true openness and emotional honesty, I had created a direct barrier to my own path of healing.

Giving myself permission to be vulnerable turned out to be one of the greatest gifts I ever gave myself. Embracing vulnerability provided me with so much clarity and enabled me to release so many burdens I had been carrying unnecessarily for so long. Sure, I had managed to carry them with apparent ease, but that didn't mean they weren't really fucking heavy! It turned out that much of what I carried wasn't even mine to bear; these burdens belonged to others, and I needed to return them to their rightful owners. I had mastered the art of disguise and skillfully hid my true feelings and authentic self under many layers of pretense and emotional armor. But now it was time to undress from this facade and begin to master the art of healing.

I did a lot of work—through literal blood, sweat, and tears. I explored and experimented with countless healing modalities, some of which were successful while others were not. Among these, I personally had the biggest breakthroughs and success with hypnotherapy. It proved to be life-changing for me.

However, the breakthrough only came after I was willing to fully surrender to being vulnerable and allowed myself to feel exposed. For years, I had kept secrets to keep others comfortable, and the thought of revealing them out loud in front of someone else terrified the shit out of me. But I had reached a breaking point and felt I had nothing left to lose. I knew that in my quest to fit in, I had already lost every authentic part of myself. So I took a leap of faith and hoped that being vulnerable would allow me to finally gain something. The results were far beyond my expectations. Speaking my truth brought forth deep healing, personal growth, and expansive change. It allowed me to reclaim parts of myself that I thought were lost forever. The process not only altered my internal landscape but also changed the trajectory of my life.

For over a year, I had followed a local girl on Instagram who was a certified clinical hypnotherapist. Her posts and success stories intrigued me, but I remained skeptical. As someone who was adept at hiding my truths, the thought of unveiling them to someone in my hometown was very unsettling. The idea of anyone other than my mother knowing my deepest, darkest secrets was terrifying. Then one day she shared something that resonated deeply with the parts of me that needed to hear them, which prompted me to immediately reach out to her for a consultation.

When my appointment time arrived, we spoke on the phone, and she patiently explained the process of hypnotherapy and what I could expect in terms of results. I was ready and didn't hesitate. Everything about this venture felt right, so I immediately purchased a package to work with her and booked the earliest available appointment. It was two weeks out, and even that felt too long because I was ready *now*. I had reached a point in my healing journey where I felt stuck and unable to move forward without delving into the deeply buried archives of my past. From everything I had heard and read, hypnotherapy seemed like the path that could help me unlock those hidden parts of myself. It felt like a leap of faith, but it turned out to be exactly what I needed to break through the barriers that had held me back for so long.

My first session with her was quite gentle. During our consultation, I had jokingly warned that she probably wouldn't be able to hypnotize me right away because I was a stubborn control freak. She laughed and accepted the challenge, but I was serious; evidently, so was she. That first session involved suggestive hypnosis, and to my surprise, she had me under her "spell" almost immediately. It felt good to surrender and trust the process, especially since those were two extremely difficult things for me to do. When we finished, she gave me a recording to listen to over the next two weeks before our next session. I diligently did my homework and listened to the recording daily, but I was anxious for the next session.

When we met again, she explained that this session would be interactive and that we would be delving as deep as my subconscious would allow. We began by addressing my feelings of fear and helplessness that were impacting me daily. I tuned into the most recent experience involving those emotions, then we traced them backwards from there. It didn't take long before I found myself face-to-face with my first physical test at the firehall. The memory was so vivid and intense that it felt like I was experiencing it all over again. I could see it, I could smell it, and I could hear it. My breathing shifted to gasps as a surge of fear and humiliation ran through my body. We remained in this space for a while and worked through every detail that was happening to me and around me. From there, we continued to delve deeper into my past as we traced the same feelings of fear and helplessness. It was a wild ride! Eventually, we reached a point where I couldn't go any further, which signaled that we had arrived at the root cause of these emotions. We had ventured into a past life regression, which was just as vivid as the previous spaces we had been from my current life.

I found myself in what appeared to be a castle. The floors and walls were made of solid rock and the atmosphere was damp and musty. I was dressed in rags and was on my hands and knees scrubbing the floor with a bucket of water and a small brush. A man was standing over me with a stick in his hand, disapproving of my actions and repeatedly hitting me. I could feel the blows as I flinched in pain and begged him to stop. My reaction only made him hit me harder. The hypnotherapist asked me if I could see a door or a way to escape. I noticed some stairs in the distance with a door at the top, but I knew I couldn't escape from the man. She then instructed me to imagine my current self entering the scene to speak to the woman on the floor. I was to tell her what I knew she needed to hear. I then confidently walked through the door as my current self and descended the stairs to where the two of them were. Ignoring the abusive man, I focused on the woman, who looked up and met my gaze. Her eyes were filled with defeat and desperation.

"Stand up!" I bluntly told her.

Her expression was filled with hesitation. I extended my hand and repeated more forcefully.

"Stand up! Stand on your own two feet! *Stand up!*"

She reached for my hand, and I helped her off the floor and led her up the stairs and out the door, slamming it shut behind us. From that point, we began backtracking and reexamining each piece that had emerged during the process going in. As I revisited each memory, I found that while they still existed vividly in my mind, they no longer provoked any emotional response.

When we returned to the scene at the firehall, I could visualize it as clearly as I had before, but the intense emotions that initially accompanied it were absent. I felt no fear, no humiliation, no sense of helplessness. Instead, I experienced a surprising sense of joy and began to laugh. The sound of the captain's laughter and the sight of his cruel smile, which had previously haunted me, now had no hold over me. It was wildly empowering to be sitting in this space and feel nothing but pity for him.

We concluded the session and were easily able to identify a recurring theme that had consistently surfaced. Every instance I had of feeling fear and helplessness was tied to encounters with men in positions of authority. This pattern had repeated itself multiple times over the course of my life and seemingly in past lives as well. Each time, I had internalized and taken ownership of their actions, allowing their authority to dominate my emotional state.

Talk about eye-opening! This realization was monumental. For most of my life, I had worked tirelessly to maintain peace by being silent and compliant. But it was never my peace that I was safeguarding! In my quest for acceptance, I had given away all my power. I had diminished myself and remained silent to avoid conflict by trying to prove that I could be trusted and was worthy of their approval. Consequently, I had suppressed my true self to prioritize others' comfort over my own and consistently downplayed my accomplishments.

Not long after my hypnotic breakthrough, I embarked on a solo road trip and found myself engrossed in a podcast. The discussion centered on how being the first to achieve something made you a legend. The message struck me with such force that it felt like a slap across the face. I had to hear it again in its entirety. Frantically, I scanned the highway for the nearest pullout, and as soon as I spotted one, I swerved off the road, slamming on the brakes. While I could admit that it wasn't the safest maneuver, the urgency was undeniable. I went to the beginning of the episode, cranked up the volume, and listened intently. As the podcast replayed, I leaned in as I listened. When it was over, I realized I was holding my breath. I exhaled deeply as I hit Pause and sat there in stunned silence. It was *me*. Holy fuck! I was a legend! I had never allowed myself to fully grasp the magnitude of my accomplishment. For so long I had downplayed my achievements, and it felt foreign to accept it at that level. But as the reality of this truth washed over me, I felt a strong sense of empowerment. It was as if I had just been reunited with a missing piece of myself. A smile spread across my face and kept growing wider until my cheeks hurt. Suddenly, my voice came to life on its own.

"I AM A LEGEND!" echoed through my vehicle.

I repeated it multiple times because saying it out loud made it feel real. For the very first time I truly absorbed the truth of being a legend and felt an immense sense of pride and power.

I achieved the milestone of being *the* first and only career female firefighter in the department and that was a distinction that could never be taken away from me. I didn't attain this accomplishment because of who I knew or from any connections—I didn't have any! There were no favors, no shortcuts, and no one handed it to me on a silver platter. I showed up, day in and day out, and poured my blood, sweat, and tears into every step of the journey. I fucking earned it through sheer determination and relentless effort. On my own, I carved this path and reached this pinnacle. *Me.* I did that!

CHAPTER 28

Resurgence

The image I believed I needed to uphold was my greatest struggle. I had become a prisoner to perfection, convinced that any deviation from this flawless facade would be a sign of weakness or failure. I didn't realize that I was allowed to evolve, to grow beyond the constraints of my self-imposed illusion. Breaking free from this illusion required me to confront the truth and dismantle the veil of perfection I had so carefully constructed. Living as a prisoner to perfection meant constantly pretending to be someone I wasn't. My life became a charade, a series of calculated moves designed to maintain a flawless image. I was trapped in a fake storyline, desperate to uphold an image that didn't reflect my true self. This relentless pursuit of perfection filled my life with lies and half-truths and created a suffocating environment where authenticity was sacrificed for appearances.

The only way out of this trap was through honesty. I had to face the reality of my experiences and embrace the messy, imperfect parts of myself that I had long tried to hide. This meant admitting to myself and others what I had been hiding: the shame I carried for the secrets I kept to protect others, and the fear of not being accepted or loved with vulnerability. I was struggling.

I needed to tell the truth. *The whole truth.*

Not just the polished version I'd allowed others to see, but the raw, unfiltered reality of my childhood, the struggles and triumphs that had shaped my life, and the experiences that had defined my career. But how would I do that after so many years of lies, deceit, cover-ups, and secrets? Where would I even start? The only place I could begin was with myself. I had to confront the truth about what I had experienced and hidden for so many years. This meant peeling back the layers of denial and facing the reality of my past with an honesty I had never allowed myself to embrace. I had to call myself out and face every past version of myself with a level of brutal honesty that was both painful and necessary.

It was incredibly hard—so fucking hard! Each revelation felt like a wound reopening, but it was through this process that I began to heal. Admitting the truth to myself was the first step in reclaiming my power and my voice. It was one of the hardest battles I've ever fought but it was also the best gift I ever gave myself. By facing my past with courage and honesty, I set myself free from the chains of my own making, allowing myself to move forward with newfound strength and clarity.

One by one, I came face-to-face with every past version of myself. First, the innocent child, who had learned too many harsh truths far too young—yet somehow, she managed to hold onto fragments of wonder. Then came the rebel, bold and fearless, who tested the limits of her world and dove into the unknown without hesitation, hungry for experience. Next was the seeker, a restless spirit driven by an unquenchable desire for more—more than the life laid out for her, more than what was expected. She was relentless in her pursuit, never shying away from challenges or the unknown, determined to carve her own path. Then there was the victim, who endured cruelty she never deserved. She wore the weight of mistreatment and trauma like armor, though it threatened to shatter her at every turn. Her heart bore scars that told stories of pain, but beneath it all remained a quiet strength. Following her was the survivor. She was forged in the fires of adversity and refused to be consumed by it. With each trial, she rebuilt herself, piece by piece, no matter how broken she felt. She may have been battered, but she was not defeated. Then appeared the giver, selfless to a fault. She poured herself into others, sacrificing her needs, her desires, and even her happiness to uplift those around her. She forgot herself in the process and found fulfillment in seeing others thrive, even though it meant losing parts of herself along the way. Finally, there stood the Phoenix, her presence commanding and serene. She was the one who had risen from the ashes of all that came before. With every hardship and every victory, she learned to embrace her scars rather than hide them. She accepted her past, faced her truths, and emerged into a newfound strength and clarity. She was a being of fire and grace, soaring with honesty and self-acceptance.

Each encounter was a moment of profound reckoning. I got down on my knees and begged for their forgiveness, acknowledging the times I had criticized, mistrusted, and lied to them. These past selves, each enduring their own struggles and triumphs, had deserved better than the harsh judgments I had placed upon them.

I slowly rose from my knees, reclaiming my power, and made a solemn vow to honor and celebrate each of these women. I promised to recognize their strength, resilience, and courage—qualities that had carried me through the darkest times. I swore to be forever thankful to each of them for their part in my journey, for without their perseverance, I would not be standing in the present moment.

With this newfound appreciation, I realized that my past wounds were not just scars but sources of powerful wisdom. These experiences had equipped me with insights and strength that I could now use to serve a higher purpose and make a greater impact. Each past version of myself had contributed to the person I had become, enabling me to transform my pain into power and my suffering into a source of inspiration for others.

I had put together all the fractured parts and integrated all the versions of myself to once again become whole. A woman of integrity, someone who truly knew her value and her worth. This transformation was not only about reclaiming my identity but about making promises to myself that I would never break.

For too long, I had been silent, my voice stifled by fear and uncertainty. The boldest and most significant promise I made to myself was to use my voice and speak my truth, no matter how uncomfortable or challenging it might be. This promise held the most meaning for me because it represented my liberation from years of suppression and self-doubt. In honoring this promise, I embraced the discomfort and vulnerability that came with it, knowing that true growth and impact often stem from the places where we feel the most exposed.

I had a story that needed and deserved to be told. My experiences, my pain, and my triumphs were not just mine to bear; they were part of a larger narrative that could inspire and resonate with others. My voice, once suppressed, has become a powerful tool for change and empowerment in the world, not just for myself, but for the countless others who might be inspired by my courage to speak their own truths.

I was experiencing a powerful resurgence, and I was fully committed to embracing it with everything I had. Stepping back into my power, I had regained my confidence and felt an incredible sense of invincibility. This wasn't just a phase; it was a complete transformation. I wasn't meant to be or do ordinary. I realized that I was made for more and achieving that required an extraordinary approach. Living a life of significance meant I couldn't move at an ordinary pace, in an ordinary setting, or settle for ordinary experiences. I needed to push beyond the boundaries of comfort and familiarity. My journey required me to face challenges head-on, to walk through the coals, to stand in the flames, to be forged in the fire.

CHAPTER 29

Reply All

It was early Monday morning, the final day of a long holiday weekend, and I was on the night shift when the tones sounded, notifying of a possible structure fire at an apartment building. Instantly, adrenaline surged through my veins at the thought of numerous residents potentially needing evacuation or rescue. My heart raced as we sped to the scene, fully aware of the stakes. Upon arrival, there were no flames or smoke visible from the outside. The captain verbally noted that only a few tenants were standing outside. This signaled that most of the residents were still inside, which instantly heightened the urgency and potential danger for everyone. We quickly made our way into the building, our senses on high alert. Inside, we discovered that the smoke was confined to just one unit on the top floor, and to our relief, there was no actual structure fire. As the immediate threat dissipated, I felt my heart rate gradually return to normal, and the intense rush of the moment gave way to calmness.

While the crews were busy extracting the smoke from the affected unit and hallway, I was assigned to check on another floor. As I entered the stairwell, I encountered a gentleman sitting on the stairs with a personal oxygen tank, clearly struggling to breathe. He had been trying to descend the stairs to evacuate but had been forced to stop and catch his breath. Recognizing his distress, I reassured him that it was safe for him to stay put. I checked his vitals and spent a few minutes talking with him to ensure he was okay. His condition seemed worrisome, so I decided to call for additional help. Knowing there was an ambulance on standby, I requested a paramedic to come and evaluate him further. This way, he could receive the medical attention he needed without any unnecessary exertion on his part. When the paramedic arrived, I introduced him to the gentleman and handed over his care so I could rejoin my crew and continue my original task.

A short time later an urgent voice came over the radio. There was so much static that the only word I could make out was "stairwell." Since I was right next to the stairwell door, I opened it to investigate. Inside, I saw frantic movement and realized that the man I had assisted earlier had just gone into cardiac arrest and was being lowered to the floor. I rushed in, dropping to my knees beside the patient, and began chest compressions immediately.

The scene was a flurry of activity. One firefighter removed the man's personal oxygen line, another grabbed equipment from the jump kit, and someone else sprinted to the ambulance for additional supplies. Amidst this organized chaos, I focused solely on performing CPR, maintaining steady compressions. A few rounds in, one of my colleagues did a check-in to see how I was doing. I was sweating profusely in my heavy gear, so he strategically removed my turnout coat while I continued the compressions, allowing me to work more efficiently.

The stairwell was cramped, with barely enough room for me to fit, making it impractical to switch out or pass off CPR duties. So, I stayed in place and performed compressions relentlessly. Every two minutes, we checked for a pulse. After several rounds of CPR, we finally detected a heartbeat. The man's color began to return; his heart was beating again!

"We did it!" I exclaimed as I leaned back, exhaling a huge sigh of relief.

The joy of bringing him back was celebrated by all, but our job wasn't over. We needed to carefully get him down the stairs, onto the awaiting stretcher, and into the ambulance for transport to the hospital. This required strategic planning, considerable strength, and unwavering determination from everyone involved. Coordinating our efforts, we navigated the tight stairwell, ensuring his safety at every step. With synchronized movements, we carefully lifted and maneuvered him onto the stretcher, taking great care to keep him stable. Finally, we transported him into the ambulance, ready for his journey to the hospital.

Once the ambulance departed, there was a palpable sense of teamwork and achievement. We exchanged mutual pats on the back and heartfelt "well done" comments. Successfully saving a life brought a deep, shared satisfaction to everyone involved.

As we walked back toward the apartment complex, we noticed several tenants still sitting outside in the entryway. Suddenly, one of them called out, informing us that he was experiencing chest pains. Instantly, my colleague and I snapped back into action. The man explained that he had been stung by a bee and being allergic to bees, was now suffering from chest pains. Recognizing the urgency of the situation, I immediately dispatched for another ambulance while we quickly assessed his vitals. We worked efficiently to keep him calm and stable while monitoring his condition closely. Fortunately, the ambulance arrived swiftly, and the paramedics took over his care. I breathed a long sigh of relief knowing both patients had received necessary treatment promptly.

As we were wrapping up our response, dispatch notified us that a grass fire had reignited in a residential area on a nearby mountain. Without hesitation, part of the crew broke away to tackle the new fire, while the rest of us completed our tasks at the current scene. Once we ensured the scene was stable and clear of any threat, we headed back to the firehall to gather additional gear before responding to the grass fire. By this time, it was late morning, and although our shift was supposed to have ended at eight a.m., our duty continued to call. The rigors of firefighting demand flexibility and readiness, and despite our exhaustion, we remained committed.

We spent several hours tending to the grass fire, working tirelessly to contain and extinguish the flames. Once the fire was finally put out, we made our way back to the firehall, eager to clean up and head home. The exhaustion hit me hard; I was both physically drained and ravenously hungry. Covered in soot and grime, all I could think about was getting out of my gear, going home to shower, and eating.

Once back at the firehall, we meticulously cleaned and stowed our gear, ensuring everything was ready for the on-duty crew and the next call. The thought of a hot shower and a meal was the only thing keeping me going. After what felt like an eternity, I was finally able to leave and head home. However, my reprieve would be short-lived. I only had a couple of hours to rest and recharge before I had to return at six p.m. for my second fourteen-hour night shift.

It had been an unbelievably hectic day but that's precisely what I loved about the job. The unpredictable nature and the constant demand for readiness and action kept me engaged and motivated. Experiencing the full scope of what it means to be a firefighter—responding to emergencies, saving lives, and protecting property—was the most gratifying aspect of the job. The events of the day had been wild, filled with intense moments and high stakes. From the adrenaline rush of responding to the initial structure fire call, to the urgent lifesaving efforts in the stairwell, and the unexpected challenge of the grass fire, every moment tested our skills and resolve. Despite the chaos and exhaustion, there was an undeniable sense of fulfillment in knowing we had made a tangible difference.

The rewards of the job came in many forms: the camaraderie with my fellow firefighters, the relief of those we helped, and the personal satisfaction of overcoming each challenge. As exhausting as it was, days like this one reaffirmed why I chose this profession. The sense of purpose and accomplishment was unparalleled and made every demanding moment worthwhile.

As a member of the social media committee, I took it upon myself to create a detailed Facebook post sharing a couple photos and the story detailing the incredible experiences and accomplishments of our crews that day. With immense pride, I documented every moment of our tireless efforts and triumphs. I couldn't help but feel a profound sense of achievement as I recounted the events. We had not only worked our asses off but had also saved a life amidst the chaos.

The intensity of the day showcased our dedication, resilience, and unwavering commitment to serving our community. I felt it was essential for the community to know what their firefighters had been up to on that seemingly quiet Monday. I wanted to spotlight the hard work and bravery that happened behind the scenes to ensure their safety. Through the Facebook post, I was able to convey the pride we felt in our work and the gratitude we had for their support.

It didn't take long for the buzz to start about the press release our boss issued following that day's events. The statement was extremely brief, merely mentioning that we had tended to smoke in a unit and a "minor medical emergency" with no further details. *Minor* medical emergency? What the actual fuck! I was surprised, but at the same time—considering the source—I was not surprised. It was well-documented in the report, and known among my peers, that I had been the one performing chest compressions throughout the ordeal and ultimately got that man's heart beating again. Yet here was our boss, downplaying the significance of our efforts and offering no acknowledgment of the lifesaving work we had done. This wasn't an isolated incident but rather a consistent theme in how our achievements were treated. I had to at least give them credit for consistency, even if it was consistently disheartening. Despite the lack of official recognition, I knew the truth about what we had accomplished. Our team had shown exceptional skill and dedication, and we had made a real difference that day.

I sat down at the computer to check my work email and opened one that had been sent to the entire department. It was a forwarded copy of the medical examiner's report regarding our calls from that hectic day. As I reviewed the report, I saw that we were acknowledged for our medical efforts and given recognition for a job well done. I sat back, staring at the screen, and reread the words multiple times, absorbing the validation we rarely received. I closed my email and told myself I needed time to process what I had read and to calm the emotions that were surfacing. I knew what I *wanted* to do, but I needed to take a moment to think it over.

That night after work I reflected on the events that had happened that fateful day, and the lack of internal recognition we had received despite our life-saving efforts. The next day, when I got on shift, I reopened my email and hit "reply all." In my response, I expressed how amazing it was for us to receive the deserved recognition, even if it only came from an outside source. I couldn't let this slide by again without saying something. Our efforts deserved to be recognized, and it was crucial to hold our bosses accountable for appreciating their hardworking people.

My mind was buzzing with questions. Why was it such a challenge for management to see the positive impact we were making for the department? When our team excelled and saved lives in the community, why didn't they seize the opportunity to highlight our efforts and showcase how dedicated their firefighters were in serving the public? Why wasn't there a sense of pride in our accomplishments, a desire to boast about our achievements? These thoughts swirled in my head as I tried to grasp the reasoning behind the lack of recognition. It seemed baffling at first. Why not celebrate and elevate your team when they were performing at their best? But then it dawned on me. It wasn't about everyone else; it was about me.

A couple of days later, I arrived at work for my first day shift and was immediately approached by a union executive member who asked to speak with me privately. He informed me that my bosses were extremely upset about the email I had sent and wanted to meet with me to discuss it. He offered me the option to address the issue with them immediately, with his support, or to take some time and have the meeting later with a different executive member. I didn't see any point in waiting, so I opted to face the situation right away. He then mentioned disciplinary action was being considered and suggested that I might want to apologize to potentially mitigate the consequences. I nodded, but internally, there was no fucking way I was going to apologize. I wasn't sorry for what I did; I stood by my decision to speak up for my team.

We made our way downstairs for the meeting. In the past, such a confrontation would have left me insanely nervous—my mouth dry and begging for water, and my voice hesitant. But not anymore. This time I felt powerful and was eager to stand by my actions and explain my motivations. We entered the office and the four of us sat down at a round table. I folded my hands neatly in my lap and remained silent, allowing them to speak first. As each of my bosses talked, I maintained steady eye contact, observing the pathetic display of authority unfolding before me. It didn't take long before there were threats of escalating the matter to HR and imposing disciplinary action. Their threats were challenged with a calm and unflinching demeanor from me.

"If that's what you feel you need to do," I responded simply, with zero reaction.

I could see the surprise in their eyes, including my union rep, who then lowered his head. I imagined they were expecting fear, or at least a reluctant apology, but I gave them neither.

In my entire career, I had never been written up or disciplined for anything. My record was spotless, and I wasn't the least bit worried. The threats didn't intimidate me as they were likely intended to. I sat there stone-faced, shrugged my shoulders, and genuinely didn't give a fuck. As each continued, they informed me that they would not be disrespected by staff taking it upon themselves to reply to emails like that. There it was! That was my window of opportunity, so I seized it.

"I'm sorry you took it that way," I said, meeting the eyes of my boss directly and watching his expressions carefully. "That's not how I intended for it to come across."

That was my half-assed attempt at an apology. It was literally the only way the words "I'm sorry" were going to come out of my mouth, so I was very careful with my wording. The truth was, I wasn't sorry at all. I had been *very* intentional when I sent that email, and I meant every word of it. My so-called apology was a strategic move, designed to address their grievances without compromising my stance. I knew exactly what I was doing, and it was essential to maintain my integrity. I was fully aware of the significance of my actions and the message I was sending.

I was then asked why I had chosen to "reply all" to the email in the first place.

"We deserved the recognition," I stated firmly. "And it was disappointing that such acknowledgment had to come from an external source. Our own leaders failed to recognize our work and downplayed it in the press release as a *minor* incident. We literally saved someone's life, and there was nothing minor about that."

One boss immediately got defensive and claimed that he hadn't referred to it as a minor incident. I held my ground.

"Yes, you did," I insisted. "You were literally quoted saying so in your press release."

He continued to deny it, suggesting that the media must have sourced the information from the firefighter's Facebook post because he had never said it.

"I wrote the firefighter's Facebook post," I claimed, looking him straight in the eye. "So I know for a fact that it didn't mention a *minor* medical emergency."

Looking anywhere but at me, he denied that his report said it was minor. My patience was wearing thin, and my frustration grew. I could not tolerate lying, so I stood firm and pushed even harder for the truth.

"Why don't we bring up both social media posts so we can compare the exact wording on both?" I suggested.

It was a simple enough task, and I reached for my phone to do it. My boss stuttered, making excuses and saying it wasn't necessary. Confident in my correctness, I reiterated that it was necessary to uncover the truth. The subject quickly shifted back to HR.

"I was thinking that involving HR might not be the best idea," one boss backpedaled. "We know how harsh she can be, so I think we'll just deal with this incident amongst ourselves."

I leaned back in my chair and crossed my arms over my chest as the heat started to rise in my face.

"You're a fucking coward!" The words echoed loudly in my head as I looked at him with disgust from across the table.

A few more things were said by them, but I had stopped listening. Disengaged, I simply waited to be dismissed. As I walked away, I found myself chuckling inwardly at the absurdity of the situation. It was a stark reminder that I was working under bosses, not leaders. The distinction between the two had always been clear to me, but this encounter solidified it beyond any doubt. It wasn't the first time I had noticed, but now it was ingrained in my consciousness, making it impossible to overlook or dismiss.

I believed deeply in what I was doing for my community, and I was immensely proud of the impact I had made. I knew the value of my work. I knew the dedication of my colleagues and the hard work we put in. We had made a significant difference, and I wasn't wrong in what I said. Despite the lack of recognition from our so-called leaders, I remained steadfast in my conviction. Given the opportunity, I would 100 percent do it again. I would continue to stand up for the truth and for the recognition we deserved. This experience, while disheartening, only reinforced my commitment to my values and my mission.

For years, I had fought my battles alone without any backup. Eventually, I gave up fighting for myself. But that time had passed. I was no longer willing to stay silent or accept the status quo. Now, I was not only speaking up and fighting for myself, but also standing up for my colleagues. I believed in their dedication and integrity, and I was determined to advocate for them just as fiercely as I did for myself. I had found my voice, and I was using it to speak the truth. My words rang louder than the lies that had been perpetuated for too long.

A few months later, I found myself strolling into a local grocery store on a bright, crisp morning. As I turned the corner just past the entrance, I suddenly came face-to-face with the gentleman whose life we had saved. My heart skipped a beat at the unexpected encounter, and a warm sense of pride and relief washed over me. The memory of that harrowing day was easily restored in my mind, and seeing him standing there, very much alive, felt nothing short of a miracle. As our eyes met, a gentle smile spread across his lips, and I couldn't help but smile back, feeling a sense of connection in that brief moment.

"Good morning," I said warmly.

A part of me wanted to say his name, as it was etched in my memory from our brief but intense encounter. But for some reason, perhaps out of a sense of respect or uncertainty, I held back. He returned my greeting with a genuine smile, and with a steady hand he continued to move along slowly, supported by his cane.

As I watched him walk away, I wondered if he remembered me and our conversation in the stairwell that fateful day. It was a question that would likely remain unanswered. But seeing him alive and clearly still recovering filled me with a profound sense of fulfillment. It was a silent acknowledgment that our actions had made a difference, which was enough for me.

CHAPTER 30

The Power of Peer Support

When I began my career in the fire department, there was a complete absence of critical incident stress management. Resources were nonexistent and the topic of mental health was never broached. After responding to a call, the ride back to the firehall was characterized by a heavy, uncomfortable silence.

"You're fine, right?" would occasionally be said to break the silence.

The expected response to the old-school statement disguised as a question was always a terse yes, and that was the end of any discussion.

Upon returning to the firehall, the teamwork that existed on the scene seemed to dissipate. Everyone would scatter in different directions, seeking solitude or distraction, and conversations about the incident were rare, if they happened at all. The culture was one of stoic endurance, where showing vulnerability was frowned upon. This created an invisible barrier that prevented us from admitting to one another how deeply the traumatic events we witnessed affected us.

Being new to the department, and perhaps because I was a female, I had a unique perspective. As a natural observer and people-watcher, I paid close attention to body language, tones of voice, and overall demeanors. I noticed how these changed after certain calls. I observed reactions filled with anger and saw the prevalence of unhealthy coping mechanisms. From the beginning, I witnessed good men being mistreated by those in authority. It wasn't just me who faced this; although my experiences were far more intense, others were also on the receiving end of such mistreatment. I saw the toll it took on them, driving some to drugs or alcohol as means of numbing the pain. While some of these vices were likely due to the traumatic nature of our work, I knew that dealing with certain toxic individuals in the workplace exacerbated the problem. We didn't get to choose our coworkers and personality clashes were inevitable. Working for three years side-by-side with toxic people or under the command of someone I could neither respect nor trust was incredibly challenging. I could sympathize with the guys placed in these unfavorable positions. I always viewed things from a different angle and understood the impact of toxic leadership. In my eyes, earning a higher rank was a privilege that came with the responsibility of leading with respect and integrity. Unfortunately, many saw it as a right, which they misused, becoming selfish and disrespectful, often trying to break good people. This misuse of power and lack of empathy troubled me and fueled my determination to bring about change.

In my first five years of being a career firefighter I saw first-hand the toll these experiences were taking on some of the men and I knew something had to be done. Determined to make a difference, I became a strong advocate for introducing critical incident stress management and peer support into the department. While some individuals frowned upon these efforts, it was undeniable that they were necessary.

Admittedly, my advocacy was partly driven by my own need for these resources. I recognized how desperately we all needed support, and I believe such measures should be a standard portion of firefighter training. It's not a question of if we're going to need it, but when. I argued that implementing stress management and peer support was essential for the mental health and well-being of everyone in the department. Firefighters face immense psychological pressures and providing the right tools to cope with these challenges was crucial. I envisioned a department where mental health resources were readily available, reducing the stigma around seeking help and ensuring that no one had to suffer in silence. This initiative was about creating a healthier, more supportive environment for all of us.

The chiefs agreed to introduce crisis intervention training that had been readily available to first responders worldwide for many years. They chose to make it mandatory that everyone in the department participate in the courses to block the negative influences that were always present. From the very start, I was convinced of the program's value and knew I wanted to be deeply involved. The content resonated with me, and I recognized its potential to make a significant impact on our department. Upon completing the courses, we faced the next step: establishing a peer support team. Without hesitation, I was the first to volunteer to lead this initiative. I was eager to take on the role, knowing it would allow me to be a positive force within the department. Leading the peer support team was not just a responsibility; it was a mission I was passionate about, and I was ready to dedicate myself fully to making a difference if they would let me.

Introducing the new program faced significant resistance, much like any change. There were loud voices vehemently opposing it, declaring that we didn't need such measures and dismissing it as foolish. Ironically, I learned that those who were the most vocal in their opposition were the very ones who needed it the most. Their resistance was rooted in a longstanding culture of sacrifice and denial. The idea of seeking help or admitting vulnerability was foreign and uncomfortable to them. However, I saw through their bravado. These were the individuals who bore the brunt of years of unaddressed stress and trauma, and their pushback was a defense mechanism against confronting their own need for support.

It took quite a while to get some of them on board. Many believed that the horrific things we had seen and dealt with were just part of the job. And while that was true, we needed to be reminded that we were still human beings who deserved support, guidance, and resources when needed. A significant barrier was the stigma of not being "tough enough" to handle the job. I felt it myself.

There was a constant pressure to suppress vulnerability, to push through without showing signs of weakness. It was as if admitting to being affected by the trauma we encountered meant you weren't fit for the role. The fear of one traumatic incident spiraling into something larger was always in the back of my mind. I worried that an event could lead to a lasting impact—an unseen brain injury, emotional burnout, or psychological distress that might leave me unable to perform, or worse, cost me the job I had worked so hard for. I knew I wasn't alone with the weight of this fear—that some of my colleagues were carrying the same burden—silently afraid that admitting to struggling would be seen as a personal failure or a professional liability.

What troubled me even more was the culture that allowed these fears to fester. We worked in environments where resilience was often measured by how well you could pretend nothing bothered you, even when it clearly did. Unlike most professions, where employees don't face the daily fear of trauma breaking them down, first responders live with this pressure constantly. For most people, the idea of a bad day at work doesn't include the risk of life-altering injury—physical or emotional— but for us, the stakes are different. I knew this unhealthy dynamic needed to change.

The unspoken rule was to endure silently. Speculations about the consequences of admitting our struggles ran rampant but no one really knew for sure because no one had ever come forward and admitted they were struggling. This culture of silence was damaging, and I aimed to break it by fostering an environment where it was safe to seek help. What worried me the most was my deep concern about how others perceived me. I questioned whether I would have the courage to openly admit to my colleagues and bosses if I was ever hurting and needed help, for fear that my vulnerability would be met with judgement instead of support.

There were aspects of the job where I witnessed and engaged in activities that most people would struggle to comprehend. We encountered horrific scenes that left indelible marks on our minds—experiences that could and did—shorten careers if not managed properly. I had always prioritized healthy coping mechanisms, which was something many of my colleagues lacked. I understood that the psychological toll of our work was immense, and without proper support, the consequences could be dire. A valued colleague quit his career, two others took mental health leaves of absence, and two acquaintances from other departments died by suicide.

I took pride in this aspect of my resilience, recognizing that effective crisis management would be crucial in supporting both myself and others. My commitment to maintaining mental health wasn't just about personal survival; it was about ensuring that my peers also had the tools to navigate the emotional and psychological challenges we faced. The introduction of critical incident stress management and peer support was, in my view, essential to sustaining our careers and well-being. My vision was to see a department where every firefighter could rely on healthy coping mechanisms and peer support to handle the darkest aspects of our job. By championing these changes, I aimed to protect not only our careers but our overall quality of life, ensuring that we could continue to serve our community without sacrificing our mental health.

For nine years of my career, I had the honor of serving as the peer support team leader. This role was one I approached with great seriousness and dedication, believing that I could make a meaningful impact—even if it was often behind the scenes in secret. It was immensely rewarding to be entrusted with supporting several of my colleagues through some of their most challenging times. Being able to serve them in this capacity meant a great deal to me. The trust they placed in me during their moments of vulnerability was a privilege I never took for granted.

My commitment to providing support and guidance extended beyond my own department, as I was often called upon to assist individuals and groups in neighboring departments as well.

Over the years, I built a reputation for reliability and empathy and became a trusted figure in the realm of crisis management and peer support. My role often required me to assist in various forms, from one-on-one support sessions to broader departmental interventions. In this role, I saw firsthand the profound difference that effective peer support could make and reinforced my belief in the importance of mental health resources in our line of work. It wasn't just about providing immediate relief; it was about fostering a culture of openness, resilience, and mutual aid. As time passed, the evolution of retirements and new hires brought in younger firefighters who were more open to the idea of mental health in the workplace. Their growing numbers gradually outpaced the negative voices, leading to an incredible cultural shift. The younger firefighters valued having support available and embraced the vision of maintaining healthy careers. They enhanced my efforts of compassion and support and jumped on board the crusade of ensuring that every firefighter knew they had someone to turn to in their darkest moments.

The passion I had for my purpose far exceeded anything I had experienced before and continually grew over the years. Recognizing that there was more I could contribute, I embarked on a personal quest to expand my knowledge and skills. I enrolled in numerous courses and training programs focused on assisting others through crisis and trauma. I completed the advanced levels of critical incident stress management and went on to become an approved instructor of crisis intervention courses. I became a certified trauma responder and even achieved international accreditation in community and workplace traumatology. I pursued all of this on my own time and at my own expense. Although the department and its members reaped the benefits of my efforts, I viewed it as my donation to their well-being. The entire purpose was to better equip myself to support and guide others through challenging times, providing them with the necessary resources and tools to cope more effectively. After witnessing numerous instances of self-destruction with drugs and alcohol, and experiencing alcohol abuse myself firsthand, I knew how desperately additional assistance was needed. Unfortunately, our organization, like many others, relied solely on an inadequate employee assistance program as the extent of our resources. I have found this to be a common issue among organizations, using such programs as a facade of support for their employees. Determined to make a difference, I continuously brought new information to the department bulletin board and sought out every free resource and option available for everyone. Although I was limited by the support options at my disposal, I did everything within my power to improve the situation.

During this period, I quietly began operating my own business—Fire Within Crisis Services Inc.—in the shadows alongside my work and personal life. Residents in my community often sought my support during personal tragedies and I guided them toward additional services beyond what I could personally provide. I have received urgent phone calls from individuals in and around my community on the brink of taking their own lives, making a split-second decision to reach out to me for help. Being entrusted in these moments of extreme vulnerability opened my eyes to the fragility of life. These experiences have filled me with immense compassion and empathy, free from judgment, for those courageous enough to seek help. I have been privileged to witness the extraordinary strength and bravery of individuals navigating their most painful times and am empowered by their resilience and demand for change in their lives. They will never understand the impact they had in my life and how much they inspired me to make the changes I needed to make as well.

CHAPTER 31

Bending the Rules

It was the fall of 2022, and I had just been passed over for a promotional position that everyone knew I wanted and, quite frankly, deserved. Throughout my career, we had all made five-year and ten-year plans, so it was common knowledge that I aimed to eventually move in the direction of fire prevention. However, there was one major obstacle: the current holder of the position showed no signs of leaving. If he planned to stay until retirement, and I would be retiring before him, then my chances of being promoted to that position seemed slim. The only scenarios in which I could get the promotion were if he left for another job or was promoted to a chief's position internally. So imagine my surprise and excitement when he announced he was leaving for a job elsewhere. Finally, my chance had arrived, and the timing couldn't have been better. This promotion would elevate me to captain's rank, which would increase my wage and my pension. More importantly, it would allow me to finish out my career working straight days with no more night shifts. The prospect of no longer working nights was a huge relief. This old girl was getting tired of the nocturnal grind and my mother was still constantly uprooting her life to stay with our son whenever my husband and I were both working night shifts. The new position would mean stability for my family and serve as the culmination of my career aspirations. It would make all the years of hard work and sacrifice worthwhile.

I eagerly embraced every educational opportunity that came my way over the years and always gave my best effort in every course. To advance within the department, certain educational requirements had to be met, so I consistently worked toward obtaining them to be prepared for promotion.

However, there was a persistent struggle between some members and the union executive regarding the pursuit of education beyond our current job level. At some point, the decision was made that promotions would be based solely on seniority, disregarding merit and suitability for the position. This approach seemed rooted in a fear that educated individuals might leapfrog others in line for promotion and revealed a lack of trust in the members. I firmly believed that no one would do that unless they were truly confident that the one being promoted wasn't a fit for the role. To me, the emphasis on seniority over merit indicated a preference for a simpler, less-effortful promotion process. I strongly disagreed with this reasoning and advocated for continuous learning irrespective of seniority.

Delaying education until it was one's turn for promotion seemed incredibly shortsighted to me. What if a member's circumstances changed, necessitating a move or a desire to work in a different department? Presenting a stagnant resume would not only be embarrassing but could also be detrimental to career progression. Utilizing employer-funded courses seemed like common sense to me but not everyone shared this view. In my opinion, prioritizing easy promotion based on seniority over merit was a flawed approach that did not serve the long-term interests of the members or the department.

The flaws in the union's approach were about to be exemplified. Due to the controlled pacing of my education, I found myself one course short when the promotional opportunity presented itself. Even though I knew the hiring would be based on seniority, I couldn't help but feel the importance of obtaining the course I needed so I was able to meet all the application requirements. Unfortunately, I soon found out that the earliest opportunity to take the required course was scheduled two months after the start date of the new position. I was determined not to let this delay hinder my chances, so I contacted my boss to explain my situation and expressed my eagerness to register for the course immediately. I wanted to demonstrate my drive and proactivity by indicating on my application that I was already registered. However, he informed me that the budget could not accommodate my enrollment at this time.

"I will pay for the course myself," I proposed as an option. "And then the department can just reimburse me when the budget allows."

I emphasized how important this opportunity was to me and my willingness to invest in my professional development. But despite my offer, my boss declined and explained that there were several other firefighters who also needed the course. To address this demand, he planned to bring the course to the firehall for everyone to attend.

"Missing that one course won't be an issue," he assured me.

"Are you sure it won't hinder my application?" I asked, seeking confirmation.

Again, he reassured me that he was sure.

The posting for the position was unusual in that it went out both internally and externally simultaneously. Typically, positions were first posted internally, and only if no qualified candidates applied would they be opened to external applicants.

Given that promotions were heavily based on seniority, a flurry of discussions broke out among us to ensure no one would inadvertently overstep. In our system, it was customary for the most senior person interested in the position to apply, which effectively eliminated internal competition. This practice ensured a clear path for the senior candidate to secure the role. After many discussions, and with a few colleagues' senior to me deciding to back out, it was collectively agreed that I would be the one to apply for the position. With a sense of excitement and anticipation, I diligently prepared my application package. I hadn't created a resume and cover letter in many years, so I worked hard at ensuring it was up to date and would exceed expectations. Proudly, I submitted it and was hopeful that my attempt at a proactive approach and my readiness for the role would be recognized.

The job posting closed after two weeks, coinciding with my vacation. While enjoying breakfast with a friend at a restaurant, my phone suddenly rang. Since I typically received text messages, and rarely phone calls, I turned my phone over to see who it was. Much to my surprise, it was my boss's number, which immediately sparked excitement between my friend and me. Anticipating good news, I took a deep breath and answered the call. Initially, the conversation was casual. He asked about my vacation and what activities I had planned. Although the chat felt odd and drawn out, I attributed it to my own anxiety and eagerness to hear the outcome of the job posting. However, my anticipation of good news was soon dashed. I was informed that the reason for his call was to deliver some unfortunate news. He explained that the job posting hadn't reached the full extent of its intended audience like they had hoped, so they were going to repost it for an additional length of time. As I listened, a mixture of gratitude and confusion washed over me. I was thankful for the update but bewildered by the emphasis on external recruitment despite my internal application. After dedicating seventeen years to the department, this decision felt like a blow.

I thanked him for the phone call, hung up, and sat there for a moment, processing the news. Slowly, the realization dawned on me. It wasn't about the logistics of the posting; it was about me. This felt like payback for various confrontations and challenges he and I had had over the years. Payback for standing my ground when he had his finger in my face. Payback for my husband's confrontation with him. Payback for challenging his dishonesty and threats. Payback for hitting "reply all" on an email and refusing to apologize for speaking out. The call had revealed more than just the status of the job posting; it unveiled years of underlying tensions and the true dynamics of how the entire process had been tainted.

In that moment, it became clear that this decision was not based on merit or organizational needs; it was driven by personal vendettas and power dynamics within the department. It was a sobering realization of the continuous unjust realities I faced and a true sign of weakness on his part, revealing a preference for control over meritocracy.

Once again, I waited for the job posting to close and the hiring process to commence. The waiting felt excruciatingly painful, especially as I received no phone calls, only radio silence from the chiefs about my application.

Unable to handle the uncertainty any longer, I turned to my union representatives for answers. What I learned was disheartening. My application hadn't even been considered because I was one course short of the required qualifications. The union approached the issue from various angles and proposed a reasonable compromise: offer me the position on the condition that I complete the course within my six-month probationary period. This probationary period was designed not only to assess my fit for the role but also to give me the option to return to my previous position as a firefighter if I found the new role unsatisfactory. The six-month timeframe was more than sufficient for me to learn the job and complete the necessary course. However, my bosses refused to allow this arrangement. Despite the union's fair efforts, they hit a brick wall. The excuse given was that "management has the right to manage," which felt like a feeble justification for their decision. The union had exhausted all options and there was nothing more they could do.

I was furious. This situation served as a stark reminder of the power dynamics at play within the department and the extent to which personal biases could influence professional decisions and overshadow fairness and reason.

Despite the union's fear of someone leapfrogging the line, their approach ultimately disqualified me from a well-deserved promotion due to educational holdbacks. The situation was further complicated by personal vendettas, which played an even larger role in my disqualification. The education requirement, which should have been manageable, became an insurmountable barrier because of these biases. This left the union in a powerless position to effectively advocate on my behalf.

Unexpectedly, we were all informed that there had been two qualified external applicants for the position I had been vying for, but one had withdrawn, leaving just one candidate to go through the hiring process. With no internal candidates being considered and only one external contender left, it was inevitable that without any competition, this sole applicant would secure the position. The entire situation felt off to me. Nothing about it made sense and it left a bitter taste in my mouth. Every fiber of my being sensed that something was amiss. The process seemed orchestrated in a way that defied logic and fairness. Despite not having concrete evidence at that moment, my gut told me that there was more to the story than met the eye.

It didn't take long, and the atmosphere was electric with chatter as word spread that the new recruit didn't meet all the necessary criteria either. I was instantly suspicious and needed to know more. How the hell did he secure the position without fulfilling all the prerequisites? With my knack for sleuthing, I couldn't resist diving into investigation mode. I began by examining the two job postings. My suspicions were immediately confirmed: the second one had undergone a subtle alteration. One of the required qualifications had been downgraded to a mere suggested qualification—conveniently, the very one he lacked. *What the actual fuck!* They had adjusted the requirements, and just like that, he magically fit the bill. The realization hit me like a ton of bricks. This was not just a minor oversight or an innocent mistake; it was a deliberate manipulation of the hiring process to favor an external candidate over me. The rules had been bent, and the playing field had been skewed, all to ensure that this guy could slide into the position without legitimate qualifications.

I had stumbled upon a bombshell and there was no way I was going to keep quiet about it. Absolutely livid, I wasted no time taking my findings straight to my union. The representative I confided in was utterly flabbergasted; he hadn't been aware of the situation at all. But when he escalated the matter to the next level, it turned out that one higher up was already in the know and had chosen to keep it under wraps. I was beyond disbelief. Well, maybe not entirely. Deep down, I had sensed all along that there had to be more to it than met the eye. Too many things just hadn't added up. This also gave me confirmation that what I had suspected all along was true: it was personal. The realization was a gut punch—a betrayal of trust on multiple levels. It cut to the core and revealed once again the extent to which the system was rigged against me. My boss's manipulation of the job posting to favor an external candidate, coupled with the union's complicity or negligence, exposed a network of deceit and highlighted a pervasive culture of corruption.

The betrayal served as a pivotal moment of clarity for me. It stripped away all the illusions I had built up over the years and revealed the true nature of the situation and the individuals involved. This was a reality I had chosen to be blind to for far too long. The veil was lifted, and I saw clearly how deeply entrenched the problems were within the department. It became painfully evident that there were no signs of improvement on the horizon. Instead, things had progressively worsened over time, and the downward spiral had become the norm, with no indications of it ever reversing course. I had long hoped that fairness and meritocracy would eventually prevail, but this incident shattered that hope. The manipulation of job postings, the complicity of higher-ups, and the union's silence all pointed to a systemic issue far beyond individual grievances. It wasn't just about one unfair decision; it was about a department that prioritized power and personal vendettas over integrity and competence.

As I reflected on the past years, I realized that each incident, each slight and overlooked injustice, had been part of a larger pattern. The signs had always been there, but I had ignored them and clung to the belief that things would get better. This moment of betrayal forced me to confront the harsh truth: the system was fundamentally broken, and those in power had it exactly how they wanted and were not interested in change. This realization was both devastating and liberating. It freed me from the false hope that had kept me tied to a dysfunctional system. I could no longer deny the toxic environment that had stifled my growth and eroded my trust. It was time to stop giving them chances and waiting for things to improve.

CHAPTER 32

They Kept Moving the Goal Posts

I made a promise to myself after being unfairly passed over for the promotion: I would no longer participate in online courses for certificates I wouldn't use. It was a waste of the department's money and a pointless endeavor for me. I had always envisioned retiring by the time I was fifty because I didn't want to be a grey-haired old lady humping a hose and working night shifts. I wanted to leave the department with plenty of life left to pursue other passions and interests. The only way I would have stayed past fifty was if I had secured that promotional position. Since that didn't happen, my retirement plans remained unchanged. I had under two years left before reaching that milestone age.

These final years would be dedicated to wrapping up my career on my own terms. I resolved to focus on the aspects of the job I still enjoyed and to prepare for the next chapter of my life. No more wasted energy on futile pursuits. I was determined to spend my remaining time in the department making the most of the skills and experience I had gained without the false hope of advancement.

There had never been any further talk from my boss about the course he had promised to bring to the firehall that he claimed everyone needed. The one course I needed for the promotion, but he couldn't find funding in the budget to make that happen for me. Suddenly, two senior members were selected for an all-expenses-paid trip to acquire the training without any immediate need for the course in terms of promotion or upcoming tasks.

Their selection was arbitrary, based solely on seniority rather than merit or necessity. It was a baffling scenario that once again highlighted the flaws in the decision-making process within the department and union. I had to laugh at the ridiculousness of it all.

There was a lot of shifting around happening at the firehall with one of our bosses now on leave for an undisclosed amount of time. That shifting included promoting the new guy hired for the position I had wanted over to a chief's position. So once again, fire prevention was open for a temporary six-month posting, with the possibility of it extending or becoming permanent. The job posting was pinned to the bulletin board. Like everyone else, I went to have a look. I stood there in front of it and all I could do was shake my head and laugh. There were no additional education requirements! Just six months prior those qualifications were nonnegotiable, and I wasn't even considered for it because I was missing one course. Now, it wasn't even a requirement! I couldn't even make this shit up! I was asked by multiple colleagues if I was going to apply for it.

"Abso-fucking-lutely not!" was my answer.

There was no way I was going to be their sloppy seconds or a part of their games.

Interestingly, the position was only posted internally, and a senior member decided to pursue it, which discouraged any other applicants. As a result of his move off the floor, I would be promoting up to the rank of acting captain. This leadership role was based on seniority and would allow me to take charge of a shift whenever the captain was off duty. Achieving the rank of acting captain would be the highest I would achieve in my career, so I was thrilled. Over the past few years, I had frequently assumed the role under the guidance of my captain and gained valuable experience and confidence in my leadership abilities. According to our contractual requirements, I needed to have been in supervised command of at least ten calls to qualify for promotion. I had significantly exceeded this requirement, which further assured me of my readiness for this new responsibility. The opportunity to lead and make critical decisions had prepared me well for the challenges ahead, and I was eager to embrace this new chapter in my career.

As the date approached for the implementation of the new changes, my boss had already sent an email to everyone, outlining who was being promoted and when. My promotion would take effect in two weeks.

Unexpectedly, we received an unusual mutual aid call that required several members to leave town to assist with a large-scale fire in a neighboring community. This necessitated a reshuffling of those of us who remained to cover for them. This reorganization positioned me to potentially lead my shift.

Fresh from days off, I arrived at work prepared and fully expecting to take charge, only to discover that another member was working the very first twenty-four-hour shift in our firehall's history instead. Since we never worked twenty-four-hour shifts, I immediately questioned this decision. I was informed that he was allowed to do so due to "extenuating circumstances." He had worked a busy night shift prior and admitted to the two of us that he was leading, that he was extremely tired. My colleague and I were very concerned and felt that he was not in the proper condition to work, let alone be in charge. I openly voiced my concerns to my boss and they were dismissed without consideration.

"Why am I not being given the opportunity to run my shift?" I questioned. "I'm well-rested and alert."

"You're not an acting for two more weeks, so you can't," he stated simply.

I took a moment to process the information because this explanation baffled me.

"So I'm not qualified today, but I will be qualified in two weeks?" I asked.

"Yes, that's correct," he confirmed.

It was deemed extenuating circumstances for the other member to work an unprecedented twenty-four-hour shift, yet the same consideration was not extended to me for taking a leadership role just two weeks ahead of schedule. No matter how hard I tried, I couldn't reconcile this discrepancy. This same member had been permitted to act in a leadership position years earlier without any certifications, as it had also been under extenuating circumstances.

I went directly to my colleague working the twenty-four-hour shift and raised the issue. I argued that a precedent had already been set by allowing him to take on responsibilities in the past without the usual qualifications. Therefore, I should have been granted the same opportunity. He didn't agree.

"It's not personal, Lynnette," he said. "It's just different."

This explanation did nothing to alleviate my frustration. As a result, I became increasingly angry and struggled to contain my temper. My patience had long since worn thin, and now my anger was reaching a boiling point, making it difficult to remain composed.

"It's always fucking personal!" I said in a raised tone. "You guys continually move the goal posts on me! And if you need to tell me it's not personal, then guaranteed it's fucking personal!"

I had to walk away because I couldn't stand being in the presence of someone who was blatantly lying to my face. To calm myself down, I started pacing around the truck bays, trying to collect my thoughts and control my anger. Eventually, I found some solace in the tool room, where I could sit and think in relative peace. As I sat there, I shook my head in disbelief. It seemed like the absurdity and unfairness would never end. Just when I thought they had reached the peak of their bullshit, they managed to surpass it yet again.

Throughout the day, I received multiple text messages from some of the guys who had been deployed out of town. They were asking how my first shift as acting captain was going and teasing me that I owed treats for the new position. They assumed I had naturally stepped into the role given the circumstances and based on what would have been the right and logical course of action. Sadly, I had to inform them that this wasn't the case. I explained that, instead of me, another member was inexplicably given the leadership role, and in the form of a twenty-four-hour shift. Their responses were unanimous in their shock and disbelief. Each one questioned the decision, reinforcing what I already knew: our department didn't operate on twenty-four-hour shifts, and I met all the necessary requirements to be in the acting position. It seemed straightforward but my boss apparently felt otherwise. They trotted out the same old bullshit line about how "management had the right to manage."

Now I was beyond frustrated, so I sought assistance from my shop steward, and we began scrutinizing the contract because I was fully prepared to file a grievance. I was advised to go higher outside of our union, so I made several phone calls and spoke with other representatives, feeling at a loss for trusted allies and uncertain about how to navigate the situation. My predicament was particularly complex because it involved not just management but also a grievance against a fellow union member. This was uncharted territory for me; I had never fought back before. But I had reached my limit and decided it was time to stand up for myself.

My shop steward and I meticulously followed grievance protocols and talked to everyone involved. When it came time to confront my boss and hear his side of the story, the experience was utterly deflating. He confidently stood by his decision to let a tired member work a twenty-four-hour shift rather than give me the opportunity to act.

"Have you even completed your ten command calls?" he questioned.

A fact he already had to have known given my impending promotion. It was clear to me right then that I was only able to rise to the level of his belief in me and there wasn't any. This realization hit hard, especially coming from someone I had honestly expected to be more supportive. It became evident that he was willing to give me a chance at the position only when he absolutely had to, but not a moment sooner. This action spoke volumes about his lack of faith in my abilities. His reluctance to support me before the official promotion date revealed more about his true feelings than any words could.

In that moment, I knew in my heart it was time to move on.

I apologized to myself for holding on so tightly and accepting the bare minimum for so long. I recognized that I had been settling and gave myself permission to elevate my standards, to accept and expect that I was worthy and deserving of the best.

Achieving the rank of acting captain was a significant milestone in my career but it also marked a turning point in my personal growth. I knew that it was time to let go of the self-imposed limitations and embrace my true potential. I had earned this promotion through hard work, dedication, and a proven track record of commitment. Now, I owed it to myself to stand confidently in my power and fully own my accomplishments.

I'd had many conversations with my husband, so there was nothing left to discuss. We had done so much personal work together that I was finally in a space of trust and security in our marriage and felt safe and supported as I moved forward. With a clear mind and a resolute heart, I sat down in front of my computer, opened a blank Word document, and confidently began drafting my retirement letter. I kept it short and sweet, getting straight to the point. Most importantly, I made sure to proudly acknowledge myself for the honor of making history as the first and only female in the department. After rereading the letter a few times, I gave myself a nod of approval and printed off a couple of copies. Feeling a mixture of excitement and calm resolve, I walked out of my office, got into my vehicle, and drove straight to the firehall to present my letter. It all happened so quickly, yet it felt like the culmination of a much longer journey. This decisive moment was not only an end but a powerful new beginning.

I wasn't even nervous like I thought I would be. In fact, I felt an unfamiliar sense of calmness. With quiet confidence, I walked into the firehall and asked to speak privately with one of my union reps. We stepped out into the truck bays, and I turned to face him.

"I'm giving my formal notice of retirement," I stated as I handed him a copy of my letter.

Initially, he seemed confused, likely thinking I was planning prematurely since my official retirement was still a year and a half away. But as he read the letter, his expression shifted to surprise. I explained that I was giving one month's working notice, after which I would be going on my holidays and not returning once they were over. He was momentarily at a loss for words, then congratulated me and wished me all the best, which brought tears to my eyes. This was the first person I was telling, which made the moment profoundly real. Some of these guys were important to me and the realization that I was leaving them behind hit me hard. I kept my words to a minimum to maintain my composure, but in all honesty, there wasn't much more to say.

From there, I headed to the office area to present my other letter to my boss. I peeked my head into his office and asked if he had a moment to chat. When he agreed, I walked in and stepped toward his desk.

"I'm giving my formal notice of retirement," I said, handing him the letter.

He looked questioningly at me and then his eyes shifted to the paper. As he read it, I pulled out a chair across from his desk and sat down. Watching the look of surprise in his eyes and then on his face was pleasantly satisfying. He looked up at me briefly and then back to the paper as if processing what he had read.

A smile spread across my face as I shrugged my shoulders and proudly said, "Plot twist!"

"Congratulations," he said. "I hope there's no hard feelings over what happened."

Those words out of his mouth solidified my reason for being there. I gently shook my head from side to side.

"No," I said with a sigh. "It's just time."

I had so much I could have said, but as tears welled up in my eyes once more, I knew that some battles were best won by choosing not to fight. The words lingered on the tip of my tongue, but I held them back. I've grown to understand that silence can sometimes speak louder and bring more peace than any argument. Restraint in this moment was my strength, and I embraced it, letting go of the urge to engage in a conflict that might only deepen my wounds.

"I have forced things my entire career, and I'm not forcing them anymore," I told him. "I forced my way in here and haven't stopped the entire time. I have done so much work on myself. I know if it didn't flow, then it didn't align, and if it didn't align, then it's not for me."

Deep down, I knew my time there had come to an end, and I felt ready for it. With a steady voice, I informed him that I was moving forward with my business ventures.

"I really hope that if the department ever needs assistance in the future, I'll be your first call," I said.

He assured me that I would be, though I remained slightly skeptical. Despite my doubts, I wished they could set aside their egos for the sake of their people, knowing that no one cared more deeply for them or was better equipped to help than I was. My commitment to their well-being had always been undeniable. Our conversation, though lacking in substance, dragged on for a few more minutes. After a firm handshake, I walked out of his office feeling like an immense weight had been lifted from my shoulders as I headed back to my vehicle.

I wasn't sure what I was expecting to feel, but the sense of calm and gratification that washed over me was unexpected. I felt an overwhelming peace with my decision and a deep sense of pride began to take root. It was as if the universe had whispered to me, confirming that I had made the right choice. I believe that not getting the promotional position was a blessing in disguise; it had kept me from being trapped in a toxic environment for more years. Everything had aligned perfectly and nudged me to finally take the leap I had long contemplated. At that moment, I knew with certainty that this was the path I was meant to take. Everything felt right in my world.

I knew word would spread like wildfire, and there were a few colleagues I wanted to tell personally. I had immense respect for them and wanted them to hear the news directly from me first. To make an impact, I sent a screenshot of my retirement letter with the words "plot twist" and then waited. Almost immediately, my phone lit up with shocked responses. Tears streamed down my face—happy tears. I felt an overwhelming sense of peace, yet it was bittersweet to be closing such a significant chapter of my life with certain people I truly admired and cared about. There were some truly great men there and I felt privileged to have known and worked alongside them.

I sent a message to our member chat forum so that everyone would hear the news directly from me and avoid any potential rumors. I wanted to make it clear that I wasn't being driven out, as I knew some might victoriously claim. In my message, I explained that I had submitted my notice of retirement and was happily leaving with my health and plans to go all-in on my business, Fire Within Crisis Services Inc. I emphasized that I had missed enough time with my son, and I was now going to have the opportunity to be a present mother and finally be able to devote my time and energy to my family as they deserved. While I was mostly truthful in my announcement and held my head high, I did leave some things unsaid. I had established nonnegotiable boundaries for myself, which included never again working alongside or under certain individuals. This decision was crucial for my well-being and safety, and I was determined to honor it. Leaving the toxic shit storm was essential to escape their manipulative and abusive ways. I didn't need to explain this to anyone but myself. Most importantly, this departure was on my terms, and I was taking control of my life to ensure a healthier and more positive future for myself and my family.

I had reached a pivotal point in my healing journey where I could no longer waste energy trying to convince others to do the right thing. I had to let them misunderstand me, as they couldn't fathom the depths of chaos I had navigated or the fires I had walked through to truly meet myself. For far too long, I had borne the weight of their projections, only to discover, through introspection and hard work, that these burdens were never mine to carry. With deep courage, I was returning these projections to their rightful owners, and reclaiming my sense of self in the process. I made a resolute decision about what I would no longer tolerate in my life and set firm boundaries that honored my well-being. This act of self-liberation marked an incredible transformation. For the first time in over a decade, I was choosing myself, breaking free from the chains of others' expectations, and reclaiming my own narrative.

CHAPTER 33

I Don't Have a Secret; I Have a Story

One word sums up how I felt after retiring: freedom. After mastering the art of survival mode for so long, it was finally time to break free and truly live. Completing my last month of work felt almost effortless, as the light at the end of the tunnel grew brighter each day. The anticipation of hanging up my uniform for good filled me with excitement and relief. I was looking forward to the journey of self-discovery that awaited me. This new chapter would be a fresh start, with an opportunity to redefine myself and embrace life with renewed vigor and purpose. I was ready to leave behind the weight of my past and step into a future where I could prioritize my passions, my dreams, and my well-being. The road ahead was uncharted, but it promised a world of possibilities, and I was eager to explore every bit of it.

I had always been an observant person, which often put me one step ahead of those around me. My keen attention to detail allowed me to notice subtleties that others overlooked and to hear the unspoken beneath the noise. I saw the inconsistencies in patterns of behavior, detected the strategic kindness that masked selfish intent, and felt the toxic, inauthentic energy that pervaded my surroundings. Manipulation was a constant presence. Words rarely matched actions. And I was frequently gaslit by those who refused to take responsibility for their deceit. It was toxic as fuck, and while I wasn't the only one who noticed or experienced it, I have been the only one brave enough to confront it openly and tell the truth.

Throughout my healing journey, I began to find my voice and speak up, although I knew I still had a long way to go. I had reached a point where I sat stagnant and couldn't level up without telling my story, but I couldn't do so while I was still employed. Now that I had given my notice and was nearing retirement, I finally felt safe to start speaking out. I began by using my social media platforms as a space for truth-telling, sharing my experiences, and adding my commentary to various stories. One day, a long-distance friend reached out unexpectedly and wanted to connect me with a friend of hers who hosted a podcast. She had no idea how much I needed this opportunity, but it became the steppingstone out of the cage I had built around myself.

During a brief phone call with the podcast host, we immediately connected. I provided a vague outline of who I was and the premise of my story, and we scheduled a date for me to be a guest on his show. After hanging up the phone, an overwhelming wave of fear washed over me, making me feel sick to my stomach. The thought of sharing my truth on a podcast that the world could hear was terrifying, but what scared me even more was the idea that the people I worked with would hear it too. I needed time to process my emotions and decipher the frantic thoughts racing through my mind.

I had been so conditioned to fear my colleagues' reactions that I found myself slipping back into an old pattern. It was a sobering realization and as soon as I recognized what was happening, anger surged within me. How had I allowed them to maintain such control over my emotions? I had reached a point where I refused to be intimidated by them any longer. Their opinions of me held no weight and I refused to bear the burden of their actions. If speaking my truth made them uncomfortable, that was their issue to grapple with, not mine. In those moments of clarity, I reclaimed the power I had relinquished for far too long. I was proud of my ability to recognize the pattern and swiftly regain my composure. It was a testament to my growth and resilience. However, it didn't erase the lingering fear of sharing my story publicly for the first time. What it did do, though, was allow me to understand that I had the freedom to choose my path and do what felt right for me. This was both empowering and liberating, affirming that I was no longer bound by the shackles of others' expectations or judgments.

On a warm July morning, I was meticulously prepared to record the upcoming podcast episode. Armed with a set of notes as a safety net, I ventured outside to our detached shop, seeking solitude to ensure privacy and an uninterrupted recording session. While my surroundings lacked any notable podcast-worthy features, the absence of video allowed me to fly under the radar. I was ready well ahead of schedule and found myself surprisingly calm. As the host dialed in, our conversation kicked off with a discussion of technical details before he reassured me that the rest would simply flow as a conversation, emphasizing that I only needed to share what I felt comfortable divulging. He mentioned that due to the backlog, my episode wouldn't air for about a month and a half. Mentally calculating the timeline, I realized I would already be retired from the department by then, which provided me with an instant sense of security.

As the podcast intro music faded, a rush of nerves hit me like a tidal wave. Holy fuck! We're doing it! My mouth and throat were instantly parched. Grasping for my glass of water, I took silent sips while the host introduced me, his words resonating through the headphones. With trembling hands and a racing heart, I introduced myself, mustering every ounce of saliva to keep my throat from drying up. My hands were gripped tightly together, and my thumbs were massaging one another for comfort.

As the interview progressed, the host delved into questions that probed the depths of my story and offered me the opportunity to share. Each word was carefully chosen as I navigated the delicate balance between honesty and self-preservation. Despite the flood of thoughts racing through my mind, I remained steadfast, refusing to let the voice of fear dictate my narrative. That familiar voice, ingrained through years of conditioning, whispered caution and urged me to people please by withholding my deepest truths. But this time, I chose to acknowledge its presence without succumbing to its influence. I recognized that it served no purpose in this moment, refusing to grant it the power to silence me any longer.

As I courageously shared fragments of my story with the host, his reaction was one of shock and disbelief. Neither of us had any prior knowledge of what the other would ask or say, so his responses were raw and authentic, serving as a profound validation of my experiences. Hearing myself articulate these experiences aloud for the first time, I was struck by the gravity of their impact. What had once seemed like a normal part of my life now sounded undeniably distressing. The host's empathy and understanding provided a comforting space for me to unravel my truths without judgment. Despite the darkness of my narrative, there was also a glimmer of hope—a powerful message waiting to be shared. Through his guidance and support, I was able to convey this message with clarity and conviction. While my story was undoubtedly difficult to share, it was presented exactly as it needed to be. It was honest, unfiltered, and ultimately empowering.

After we wrapped up the recording, our conversation flowed effortlessly and lingered on the weight of the stories I had shared. The host's gratitude for my openness was palpable as he acknowledged the power of my message. He revealed that he intended to share our unfiltered conversation with his daughter, who aspired to become a firefighter. His desire for her to hear the unvarnished truth mirrored my own hope—that by exposing her to the realities of my experiences, she might navigate her own path with greater awareness and resilience. His words touched me deeply and offered a glimmer of hope that our dialogue could serve as a beacon of insight and inspiration for the next generation. By motivating connection through the deep unspoken bond of womanhood and drawing strength from our shared experiences, we could benefit collectively in overcoming the common traumas we face.

As we bid each other farewell and hung up the phone, I couldn't help but feel a sense of lightness wash over me. It was as though by laying down the weight of my experiences, I had shed some of the burdens I had carried for so long. As I walked back into the house, a smile played at the corners of my lips while quiet optimism stirred inside of me.

After tidying up the items I had brought out to the shop, I settled into a chair for a moment to comprehend the surreal feeling of having just been a guest on a podcast. I attempted to replay our conversation, but despite my best efforts, certain details of our discussion seemed to elude my memory. A creeping sense of panic began to take hold as I questioned the extent of my disclosure. Had I revealed too much? Could my words come back to haunt me? Were people going to be mad at me? The fear of potential repercussions loomed large, casting a shadow of doubt over my every thought. Before I knew it, I was no longer sitting and found myself pacing while impulsively straightening and cleaning random objects. It was only when I paused to take stock of my actions that I realized I needed to stop what I was doing and step outside. Even though it was warm, I put on my coat and ventured out onto the front step. The breaths of fresh air began to soothe my troubled mind. I removed my socks and descended the steps onto the grass to ground myself in the present moment.

It didn't work. I wasn't present at all. Instead, I had convinced myself that I could simply call the host and ask him for a copy to review before it aired. This way, I could ensure that nothing was included that I didn't approve of. If the recording turned out poorly, I planned to tell him we wouldn't air it. In my mind, that solution seemed perfect. It gave me a sense of reassurance, as if I had regained some control over the situation. With that matter seemingly resolved, I was able to continue with my day without giving it another thought.

The next day, I received a phone call from the host, and it felt like my worst nightmare had come true. He said he found the episode incredibly powerful and believed it needed to be heard right away. He asked for my permission to bump it up in the queue and air it the following week. From the moment he started speaking, I was completely consumed with fear. The voice in my head was screaming, *No!* But I knew, to the depths of my soul, that it was necessary for this episode to go out as soon as possible. With a shaky voice, I agreed to let him move forward with airing the podcast. The minute I hung up the phone, I thought I was going to vomit. I could feel my face flushing and sweat began to seep through my pores as panic rose within me. I immediately started to calculate the release date against my work shifts and realized I would be working my last night shift just two days before the episode would air. While it was a relief to know I'd be free from work responsibilities, I knew I needed to make plans to leave town.

Here I was, a grown woman, terrified of speaking my truth. This fear was precisely why I had decided to do this in the first place. I was exhausted from living in fear, suffering in silence, and not being true to myself. I had finally gathered the courage to leave the toxicity behind and heal myself so I could speak out and stand in my truth. No matter how far I had come, it was still incredibly scary, and I needed to grant myself the space to process the fact that others were going to hear my story.

I planned to leave town right after finishing my last shift. I wanted to be far away when the episode aired and give myself the time and space to deal with the flood of emotions and reactions that would undoubtedly follow.

CHAPTER 34

The Final Countdown

The last two weeks of work flew by. Each shift was a blend of familiar routines as I immersed myself in the tasks and calls of duty, I had come to know so well. I genuinely enjoyed the time I spent on shift and took pride in the final calls I participated in. I anticipated a wave of sadness to hit me as my departure grew closer, expecting to feel the weight of leaving behind a significant chapter of my life. But that sadness never came. Instead, I felt a sense of peace and readiness. The absence of sorrow was a clear signal to me that I was prepared to embrace this next phase of life.

It was my last night shift, and I was greeted with an outpouring of love and support when I arrived. The firehall was adorned with a variety of cards and treats that had been dropped off before I got there. Throughout the evening, many friends stopped by, bearing gifts and offering heartfelt farewell wishes. It was an incredible experience, and I felt truly blessed to be so acknowledged and appreciated by my colleagues, friends, family, and community members. As a special gesture, my captain treated our crew to supper and dessert. We feasted until we were ready to burst, enjoying every bite. The evening was filled with laughter, engaging conversations, and even a few moments of reflection on the times we had shared. The camaraderie and warmth I felt that night was overwhelming, and I couldn't have asked for a better way to spend my final shift. It was a perfect ending to a significant chapter in my life, surrounded by people who had become like family to me.

In the morning, all the members of the department arrived for a special "ring out" ceremony, a cherished tradition that leaves a lasting impact on everyone who experiences it. This time-honored ritual marks the end of a member's last shift in a memorable way. At the heart of the ceremony, the bay doors are opened, allowing the fresh air to mingle with the familiar scents of the firehouse. The members, with solemn yet celebratory expressions, climb into their respective fire trucks. The power switch makes the trucks come to life, followed by the climactic moment: the simultaneous flashing lights and blaring of sirens and airhorns fill the air with a thunderous salute to the years of service and dedication. It is a signal of the end of a watch: a heartfelt sendoff, a tribute to a career dedicated to service, bravery, and countless memories that have been forged within those walls.

I was descending the stairs when the sound of the sirens and airhorns started, bringing an instant smile to my face. The powerful noise echoed through the firehall, filling me with a mixture of pride and nostalgia. I made my way through the bay and out onto the ramp, stepping into the morning light to friends holding a banner and cheering for me. My heart exploded!

I walked to the middle of the ramp and turned to face the trucks. Their lights flashed and created a dazzling display of red and white against the dawn light. The sirens and airhorns of all the trucks blared simultaneously, filling the air with a powerful, resonant symphony. The sound was deafening yet exhilarating and it brought tears to my eyes. But these were tears of joy and fulfillment, reflecting the depth of my emotions. In that moment, everything I had been through and everything I had accomplished felt undeniably worth it. I placed my hands over my heart for the final tones, feeling the weight of this farewell. Then, with a gesture of gratitude and affection, I raised my hands to my lips and blew a kiss to my brothers. I raised my hands higher into a wave to everyone before turning and walking back into the firehall. As I moved away, the sound of the final siren slowly faded into the distance, leaving a powerful silence in its wake. It was a silence filled with memories, achievements, and the bonds that had been forged over the years. All was quiet now and I felt a sense of peace and closure as I took my last steps into the place that had been my second home.

I took a deep breath as all the guys started to surround me at the back of the truck bays, their faces filled with warmth. They wished me well, extended congratulations, and urged me not to be a stranger. The air felt thick with emotion as I shared my final moments with them. A few extended their hands for a handshake, but I waved them off.

"I don't shake hands," I said with a smile. "I'm a hugger."

I pulled each one into a heartfelt embrace, not allowing them to get away with just a measly handshake. These were the people I had trusted with my life, and a hug felt like the only appropriate way to say goodbye. There was, however, one man I left at a handshake. Our relationship had always been distant, and a handshake seemed fitting to maintain that boundary.

"I expected there to be more tears," one of the captains teased with a smirk.

In all honesty, I had anticipated a much more emotional farewell too. Instead, I felt a bubbling excitement coursing through me. This wasn't a moment of loss. I had grieved the loss long before I chose to walk away. This was now a moment of transition. It felt so right. I realized that my lack of tears wasn't a sign of indifference. Rather, it was a testament to the peace and readiness I felt about moving forward. This was a new beginning, one that I had worked hard to reach, and I was ready to embrace it with open arms.

We moved our gathering upstairs to cut into the retirement cake they had ordered for me. I felt a mix of celebration and nostalgia as we transitioned from the ceremony to this more intimate setting. As we gathered around the table, I took a moment to admire the cake, its decorative topping capturing the significance of this milestone.

In bold red icing, the cake read, "Congratulations on your retirement, Firefighter Fritshaw."

Seeing my name paired with the word "retirement" brought a smile to my face. It had always seemed like a distant milestone, something far off in the future. But here it was, unfolding right before my eyes. I picked up the knife and made the first cut, marking this moment in history.

It was early in the morning to be indulging in a slab of cake, but everyone did their best to enjoy it. I couldn't help but chuckle to myself as I struggled to eat it for breakfast. The light conversation around the table felt a little awkward at times, as if we were all trying to prolong the inevitable ending. Finally, I decided it was time to bring the gathering to a close. I stood and thanked everyone for coming, expressing my heartfelt gratitude for their presence and the cake. After a few repeated goodbyes and lingering hugs, I grabbed my things and made my way to the exit. As I walked out of the building for the last time, I felt a deep sense of contentment and readiness for what lay ahead.

I did it! I really did it.

A smile spread across my face as I put my car in reverse and backed out of my parking stall. It felt good to be driving away and leaving it behind.

CHAPTER 35

The Freedom I Deserve To Tell My Story

I had completed my last day of work, and the podcast would be airing soon. Panic surged through me, alerting me to leave town immediately. I told myself that leaving would make me feel safe, but it also stirred up a deep sadness. It was disheartening to realize that in order to feel secure while speaking my truth, I felt the need to flee. My trust in people had eroded over time, and I had learned to promptly remove myself from potentially unfavorable situations. But then, as quickly as I had panicked, I acknowledged that I had fallen into an old pattern of thinking again. I reminded myself that I was safe and had every right to tell my story. My story needed to be heard, and people deserved to know the truth. More importantly, I needed to tell the truth. This was a moment of growth, and it was time to stand firm and embrace the power of my own voice.

I did leave town, framing it as a holiday getaway with my son. Taking trips in the summertime was normal for us, so it felt like I was maintaining some semblance of routine. I received the notification that the podcast episode had aired the moment I reached my destination. Immediately, I felt a rush of anxiety and started pacing. Reluctantly, I shared the link to the episode in my social media stories and began waiting for feedback, whatever it might be. The episode was almost an hour long. Realistically, I knew it would take time for responses to come in. However, my nerves had me expecting immediate reactions. I found it impossible to concentrate on anything else and found myself continually checking my phone in case I missed a message or a text. My anticipation was palpable, and the minutes seemed to stretch into hours as I awaited the world's response to my truth.

Within the hour, messages started pouring in. My knees felt weak at the sight of the notifications, and I had to find a place to sit down. I discovered a quiet corner outside and began opening the messages. Each one was filled with words of encouragement, support, and thanks for sharing my story. Complete strangers reached out, many of them revealing that they had experienced similar struggles. Because of my story, they were feeling hopeful for the first time. As I read through each heartfelt message, I found myself in tears, moved by the genuine connections I was making. I spent most of the morning responding thoughtfully to every message. The impact of my story was profound, and it sparked conversations with so many people who felt seen and understood for the first time. Never in my wildest dreams had I imagined this outcome. I felt an overwhelming sense of pride for having the courage to speak my truth on the podcast. It had achieved exactly what I had hoped for: bringing light to a broken culture and offering hope and connection to others. And this was only the first day!

Messages continued to pour in over the next few weeks, including a concerned email from the city's human resources department with the subject titled "sexual harassment concerns." The body of the email claimed she was very disheartened to learn of my experiences after listening to the podcast. She wanted to meet to ensure that anyone who participated in harassment or who covered up bad behavior and was still employed with the city would be dealt with, and to ensure that the experience I related wasn't something that would be repeated in the future. Initially, I felt angry that they had used the term "sexual harassment," since I had never indicated anything of the sort. Then I felt hesitant and distrustful. My boss had often portrayed her as a ruthless and heartless figure, using her as a threat; so I didn't respond immediately. I needed time to process the email and consider very carefully what my response would be.

After some reflection, I decided to address the issue head-on. I sent a reply agreeing to meet but requested that we do so outside of the office. There was a lot I wanted and needed to say, and I felt more comfortable in a neutral setting. We scheduled a time, and shortly thereafter the HR representative and I met on a patio at a coffee shop. It provided a perfect balance of privacy for our conversation while still being in a public space, which made me feel safer and more at ease.

As we sat down, the atmosphere was both tense and anticipatory. She began by thanking me for agreeing to meet with her and expressed how genuinely horrified she was to learn about my experiences through the podcast. Her concern seemed sincere, but I remained guarded, listening carefully to her words. There was a brief pause, and I seized the opportunity to speak. It was crucial to address the misconceptions head-on. I took a deep breath and began with what I felt was most important: correcting the misunderstanding about sexual harassment.

"Bullying, discrimination, misogyny, and harassment, yes," I told her firmly. "But *never* anything sexual."

She quickly responded with understanding, explaining that "sexual harassment" was just a blanket term they used. But she made a note to remove it at my request. I acknowledged their concern and clarified that I understood why they had reached out, but I felt it was too little, too late. I couldn't hide my annoyance as I pointed out that no one had ever thought to check on me during the years I was enduring these issues. I knew some men in power at the time were aware of the mistreatment and turned a blind eye—speaking up would have only made things worse. Many of the current city staff hadn't been around long enough to understand what I had gone through, or even had cause for concern. I understood how my retirement and public statements pushed them to intervene, but it didn't ease my frustration. I told her plainly that I didn't need saving now, and there was nothing that could be done to change what had happened to me.

She understood my stance and apologized for their tardiness. She continued with wondering if an investigation needed to be conducted within the fire department. Most of the offenders had already retired, or were off on leave, and I felt that investigating at this point would be unnecessary and unproductive. I assured her that I wasn't seeking retribution and had no intention of naming names. I didn't need to. It wouldn't take a rocket scientist to figure out who some of the men were and I was very comfortable leaving them to their own shame and karmic repercussions.

"What I do want, though, is to be left alone to tell my story without any interference," I explained. "I want the opportunity to tell the truth about my experiences from my perspective. I believe I deserve that."

I explained to her that I had left my career specifically to gain the freedom to speak openly about my experiences and I didn't want anyone to take that away from me. She understood and agreed, assuring me that I would be given the space and freedom I needed, and there would be no further pursuit within the department regarding my past.

I continued by emphasizing that there was one crucial issue that needed attention: the future of women in the department.

"I urge you to look after any women in the future who join the department," I stated. "They deserve a proactive approach to ensure that they never have to go through what I did."

I wanted them to create a safer environment where women could thrive without fear of bullying or misogyny. I knew of many women who had been embraced and supported in building successful careers across various fire departments, and believed this should be the only acceptable experience.

"If anything positive can come from my experiences, it should be that other women can safely climb the ladder after me."

She nodded, acknowledging the importance of my request, followed by a promise that it would be fulfilled.

The conversation turned out to be highly productive and insightful for both parties involved. I gained clarity on several questions I had about the fire prevention position I wasn't even considered for. To my pleasant surprise, I discovered that my union executives had indeed advocated vigorously on my behalf and explored numerous strategies to try to secure the position for me. Additionally, I received confirmation that my bosses had steadfastly refused to consider my application and actively opposed it at every turn. This validated my suspicion that their rejection was entirely personal. Despite knowing there would never be formal consequences for their actions, I've found peace in the belief that karma has a way of balancing the scales. I wish them nothing but the days they deserve.

Everything had unfolded perfectly, positioning me exactly where I needed to be. Staying longer in that toxic environment was never part of my intended path for career growth. Instead, I was purposefully redirected, and I am deeply thankful for how it all aligned. I had endured and learned everything necessary to bring me to my current position. It felt incredibly liberating and empowering to be in harmony with my greater good, knowing that every event had occurred precisely as it was meant to.

Some of my so-called "brothers" disowned me for speaking up and telling the truth. By revealing the secrets they believed should remain locked within the walls of the firehall, I broke an unspoken code that prioritized silence over integrity. To them, loyalty meant protecting the image of the brotherhood, no matter the cost. For so long, I carried the weight of that worry, choosing silence over confrontation, attempting to maintain the bond we clearly never shared. I have come to realize that no matter how long I remained silent, no matter what I said or what I did, their decision to disown me was ultimately their own. It was not contingent on my actions but on their unwillingness to accept the truth.

Their choice to sever ties was inevitable because I chose to no longer conform to the decisions they wanted me to make. I would never again compromise my integrity to fit their expectations. They would have to own their decisions, just as I must own mine. I choose to embrace the truth and liberate myself from the shackles of secrecy.

CHAPTER 36

Notice Those Who Show Up for You

After retirement, it's a cherished tradition that the retiree is presented with a personalized wine bottle and a commemorative axe from the brotherhood/sisterhood of the fire department. These tokens of appreciation symbolize the camaraderie and respect held for those who have dedicated their lives to serving others.

I knew it would take time to order and engrave the axe, and to create the custom labels for the wine bottles. Each detail needed to be perfect to honor the retiree's years of service. The engraving on the axe would include their name, rank, and years of service. This axe wasn't just a tool; it was a symbol of strength, bravery, and the countless lives saved and protected.

The wine bottles were equally special. One bottle, with its custom label highlighting the retiree's accomplishments, would be displayed prominently in the cabinet upstairs at the firehall. This tradition allowed current and future firefighters to see and remember the legacy of those who had come before them. The other bottle would be given to the retiree to do with as they wished, whether to toast their career, share with loved ones, or keep as a memento of their time with the department.

These gestures were more than mere formalities; they were heartfelt expressions of gratitude and recognition. They honored the retiree's bravery, commitment, and the sacrifices made over the years. They also served as a reminder that, even in retirement, the bond with the fire department family would remain strong and enduring.

It had been about a month and a half since I worked my last shift when I received a message from one of my colleagues—a man who had become a cherished friend. He asked if I would be home the following morning because he wanted to stop by with a few friends. His request left me feeling both confused and suspicious, but he jokingly insisted I not ask any questions, so I complied.

The next morning I found myself anxiously awaiting their arrival. My curiosity piqued when I heard the unmistakable sound of a fire truck pulling up in front of my house. Opening the door, I saw additional personal vehicles parked and a small group of my former colleagues making their way up my driveway, accompanied by the on-duty crew from the fire truck. They came bearing gifts.

We gathered in front of my house, and one of my colleagues gave a small but heartfelt speech. His words were filled with gratitude, admiration, and respect for my years of service. They presented me with the commemorative axe and personalized wine bottle. As they handed me these meaningful gifts, I felt emotions stirring inside me. Pride, nostalgia, and a deep sense of appreciation washed over me. It was a poignant moment, not just because of the tangible tokens I received, but because of the love and respect they represented.

The axe was stunning—gold-plated and mounted in a beautiful wooden box frame. Its mere presence filled me with immense pride and held profound significance for me. The engraving read, "Acting Captain Lynnette Fritshaw, 14 years of service, 2009–2023." Achieving retirement at that rank added immense value to my career and brought a deep sense of accomplishment. It wasn't the top rank of captain, but it was close enough to feel incredibly rewarding. It meant exactly what it needed to mean to me, and that was all that mattered.

The wine bottle also carried special significance. I had chosen the picture for the label well in advance, the same image that adorns the cover of this book. Knowing exactly what I wanted, I sent the photo to the committee even before I finished my last shift. This proactive step elicited some laughs among my colleagues because there was often a delay in producing the wine bottles due to people not submitting their photos on time. But not with me. There's something to be said for a woman who knows what she wants.

The axe and wine bottle were the perfect finishing touches to my firefighting career. They encapsulated not just the years of hard work, dedication, and sacrifice, but also the respect and camaraderie that defined my time in the fire department. The axe symbolized the strength and resilience I had developed; the wine bottle, with its personalized label, was a celebration of the journey I had taken and the person I had become.

What made the day even more perfect were the six out of seventeen men who showed up for me. Their presence at my home was a profound gesture that didn't go unnoticed. They took time out of their busy schedules to honor me, and it made the occasion incredibly special. They may never fully understand how much their support and display of integrity meant to me, but I was deeply grateful. Conversely, the significant number of men who didn't show up also didn't escape my notice. Their absence was meant to make a statement, meanwhile all it did was confirm what I already knew. I also never received any farewell communication from one of my bosses—but frankly I neither needed it nor wanted it. I chose not to give any attention to the absentees and instead focused on those who were present. Their willingness to be there, to share in this milestone, was what mattered most.

The ones who came demonstrated the true meaning of the brotherhood and sisterhood. They stood by me not just as colleagues, but as friends who valued our shared experiences and the bonds we had formed over the years. As I looked around at the familiar faces, I felt a swell of gratitude. These were men who had been with me through thick and thin, who had shared in the highs and lows of our demanding profession. Their presence was a fitting tribute to the end of one chapter and the beginning of another, made all the more meaningful by the people who chose to be part of it.

CHAPTER 37

The Coolest Job In The World

Firefighting was the coolest job in the world to me, filled with countless aspects that I absolutely loved. An exhilarating, rewarding, and noble profession centered around selflessness, where I was willing to risk my life to save others and had the honor of protecting my community from harm. The adrenaline rush that accompanied rushing into dangerous situations was unlike anything I had ever experienced. Each day brought new challenges and the opportunity to make a tangible difference in people's lives. Whether it was rescuing someone from a life-threatening situation, providing comfort in their darkest hours, or preventing harm from befalling my community, the sense of purpose and fulfillment was unparalleled.

The goal was for everyone to be safe, but emergencies were when I truly got to do my job. Whether it was a fire, a motor vehicle incident, a medical emergency, or even just alarms ringing, these situations were my playground. These were the moments when my role was inherently empowering and the fulfillment that came from helping others during their most vulnerable moments was immensely rewarding. I could see the sense of relief wash over people when they realized that help had arrived. I took great pride in being one of those individuals who provided that crucial assistance. Each emergency not only tested my skills but also reinforced my commitment to serving and protecting my community. It was in these critical moments that I felt most alive, knowing that I was doing what I loved and making a real impact.

Being part of a small department meant I got to do everything. I had the opportunity to drive every apparatus, operate every pump panel, use every piece of equipment, and assume every role—from dispatcher to command. This comprehensive experience was incredibly rewarding because it ensured constant variety and kept the job exciting. No two days were ever the same. Each shift brought a new set of challenges and surprises—and a sense of mystery about what the day would entail. Every time the tones went off, it signaled a different kind of emergency, whether it was a fire, a medical call, or a rescue operation. This unpredictability prevented the job from becoming monotonous and made each day unique and engaging. Of course, there were quieter days when calls were sparse. During those times, I had to get creative with training, find tasks to keep busy, or simply kick my feet up in a recliner once everything was done and the city was safe. These slower moments, while less frequent than one might expect, were a welcome perk of the job. They provided a necessary balance that allowed for rest and recovery amidst the fast-paced, high-stress, and high-adrenaline times.

I underwent extensive training to develop a wide range of skills in firefighting techniques, equipment operation, vehicle extrication, rope rescue, emergency medical care, hazardous materials response, firefighter survival, wildland firefighting, leadership, incident command, and much more. This rigorous training ensured that I was always prepared to handle any situation that might arise, whether it was battling a fierce blaze, providing life-saving medical assistance, or managing a complicated rescue situation. These abilities became indispensable resources in my personal toolbox and equipped me to handle a variety of challenges with confidence and competence. Without my career in firefighting, I would never have mastered these crucial skills that have enriched both my professional and personal life.

Driving a fire truck code 3—lights and sirens—had to be one of the coolest and most exhilarating parts of my job. Being entrusted as the driver held significant responsibility as I navigated through traffic, maneuvered around obstacles, and aimed to arrive at the emergency scene quickly and safely. The rush of high-speed driving, combined with the need for quick decision-making and intense focus, created an unparalleled experience. With flashing lights and a blaring siren, I was not just another vehicle on the road; I was demanding the right of way. Watching as cars pulled over to clear the path, like the parting of the sea, was a powerful moment that signified both the importance of our mission and the respect from the public. Being able to drive a fire truck to an emergency is a unique privilege that most people never get to experience. The blend of responsibility, adrenaline, and public service is something I highly recommend to anyone who has the chance. An added note of caution: having that kind of power on the road is addicting. I often expected to have it in my personal vehicle as well. When road rage creeped in, my husband reminded me on more than one occasion that my car does not have lights and sirens, therefore people do not need to move out of my way.

As a female firefighter I was able to challenge traditional gender roles and stereotypes, proving that bravery, strength, and resilience are not confined to one gender. I aimed to inspire other women and girls to pursue their dreams, regardless of societal expectations, and showcase that women are valuable in positions of strength, leadership, and heroism.

The job was extremely physically demanding and mentally stimulating, providing constant challenges that required problem-solving, quick thinking, and adaptability. This kept the work exciting and dynamic for me.

Being a firefighter was a unique blend of adrenaline-pumping action, meaningful service to others, lifelong learning, and a strong sense of community. It wasn't just a job to me; it was a calling. The role demanded a commitment to serving others and making a positive impact on society. Every day brought new challenges and opportunities to learn, whether it was mastering the latest firefighting techniques, understanding complex safety protocols, or honing the physical and mental skills required to perform under pressure. This constant growth kept the work engaging and fulfilling. The respect and admiration I received from community members further amplified my sense of pride and ownership in my profession. Seeing the gratitude in their eyes, hearing their words of appreciation, and knowing that my efforts made a tangible difference in their lives reinforced my dedication to the job. Being a firefighter was more than a career; it was an expansive journey of growth, service, and connection. It shaped so many parts of who I am and instilled in me values that I carry with me every day.

CHAPTER 38

The Fire Within

Many have questioned why I remained in the fire department for as long as I did with the challenges and hardships I faced. Trust me, I asked myself that very question countless times, and the answer was always the same: I stayed because I believed I deserved to be there. I had endured failures, made sacrifices, pushed myself harder, and lasted longer than some hoped or expected. To me, this meant that I had earned my place in the department. What should have been the burning question was not why I stayed, but why it was deemed acceptable for them to treat me the way they did, even once. The adversity and abuse I endured were not things I deserved. My commitment and perseverance were met with undue hardship, which was the real injustice. Despite the manipulation and mistreatment, my dedication never wavered. I lost sight of my value but never my right to be there. It was grounded in my hard work and relentless effort. In staying, I hoped to be part of the solution, to bring light to these injustices, and to pave the way for a more equitable and respectful environment. I deserved to be there not despite the challenges, but because of my actions and my contributions. And no one deserved to endure the mistreatment I did, which is why my presence and persistence were as much a statement of resilience as they were a call for change.

I obviously stood out from the rest, but that meant I brought a unique perspective to the department, the team dynamic, the "boys club," and the broader community. My presence introduced something essential, though most were not ready to acknowledge it yet. The change I represented was inevitable and necessary and someone had to pave the way. That someone turned out to be me. For reasons beyond my understanding, I was chosen to confront the task of breaking down barriers and dismantling stigmas. It fell upon me to challenge the narrow-mindedness of many and to create an opportunity for women to find their place within the fire department. I embodied the change that this institution needed, regardless of whether they would openly admit it or not. My contribution went beyond mere presence; it was about initiating a transformation that had long been overdue. I brought a new energy, fresh ideas, and a different approach that enriched the department. It was a significant step toward inclusivity and equality, setting the stage for future generations of women to join and thrive in the fire service. My journey was about more than just fulfilling a role; it was about reshaping a culture and opening doors that had previously been closed. Whether recognized or not, I was the catalyst for this necessary evolution.

In truth, I needed that place as much as it needed me. I could have done without the manipulation and abuse, but the experiences were essential in shaping me into the woman I was destined to become. The challenges I faced were unwelcome but necessary. They pushed me to become bolder, wiser, and more powerful. Without the adversity, I wouldn't have fully grown into my potential. The struggles refined my character, teaching me resilience and strength that I might not have discovered otherwise. My journey wasn't just about enduring hardship; it was about transforming those trials into lessons. The experiences, both good and bad, were crucial in my development. They helped me evolve from a person with potential into a leader with purpose.

None of the physical abuse I experienced in my life—from the excessive spankings I received as a child to being pinned to a wall with a man's hand around my throat as an adult—none of it had the devastating impact that the psychological and emotional abuse did. The manipulation, betrayal, gaslighting, bullying, and harassment were incredibly difficult to endure. These forms of abuse deeply affected me and fundamentally changed who I was. In comparison, physical abuse felt easier to cope with. I could often defuse physical confrontations verbally or take the blame to make them stop. But with psychological and emotional abuse, there was no simple way out. I couldn't talk my way through it or shoulder the blame to make it end. The only strategy I had was to compartmentalize the pain and move on. I meticulously packed away each traumatic experience into tight, locked boxes, tucking them out of sight. They were never out of mind, but I managed to keep them hidden from others. I believe I concealed them well for a very long time.

The insidious nature of psychological and emotional abuse meant that it lingered, continuously gnawing at my sense of self. Unlike physical wounds that heal, the scars from emotional and psychological trauma remained, affecting my thoughts, behaviors, and relationships. I was in a state of constant vigilance, never able to fully relax or let my guard down. Trust became a rare commodity—I questioned everyone's motives and struggled to let anyone get close. Internally, I battled an unrelenting cycle of negative thoughts, where self-doubt plagued my every decision. I second-guessed myself at every turn, unsure whether I was making the right choices or simply setting myself up for more pain. Conflict became something I feared deeply, so

I bent over backward trying to keep the peace, prioritizing everyone else's happiness over my own, all in a desperate attempt to avoid further emotional turmoil. It was a silent struggle without visible evidence for others to see or understand. The effort to maintain a semblance of normalcy despite this internal turmoil was immense. I became adept at masking my pain and presenting a facade of strength while privately grappling with the lasting effects of it all. This concealment became a survival mechanism, a way to protect myself from further harm and keep on functioning in my daily life. Yet the cost of this internalized pain was high. It influenced my interactions, eroded my confidence, and shaped my worldview in ways that physical abuse never could. The psychological and emotional torment created a persistent shadow, a burden that I carried with me, that impacted every aspect of my existence.

I could have let what happened destroy me. The trauma and adversity knocked me down completely, leaving me in a state of despair for a long time. There were many moments when I doubted whether I could ever rise above it. I felt utterly hopeless, devoid of will and desire, teetering on the edge of giving up. The idea of quitting seemed like the only way to end the relentless torture. It would have been easy to abandon my struggles, to return to hairdressing and running my own business. That path promised peace and freedom, which was a stark contrast to the chaos I was enduring. However, I realized that giving up would have taught me nothing. It might have brought temporary relief, but it wouldn't have allowed me to grow or understand my true strength. As tempting as it was to escape, I knew deep down that quitting was not an option. It wasn't in my nature to give up, no matter how appealing it seemed.

Enduring the hardships tested me in ways I never imagined but it also revealed a resilience I didn't know I possessed. I learned that true growth often comes from the darkest moments and it's in those times that our resolve is truly tested. The easy path, while appealing, wouldn't have led to the self-discovery and empowerment that I ultimately gained. Staying the course, despite the overwhelming urge to quit, allowed me to uncover strengths and capabilities that were previously hidden. It taught me the value of perseverance, the importance of resilience, and the power of inner strength. In retrospect, I see that my decision to keep fighting was not only about surviving; it was about thriving and transforming my pain into power. By refusing to give up, I proved to myself that I was capable of enduring and overcoming even the most formidable obstacles.

People who understood my struggle often thought they were helping by telling me that if I quit, then the guys would win. Their intention was to motivate me to stay, tapping into my competitive nature and acknowledging how hard I had worked to earn my place. However, for me, it wasn't about competition or winning. I knew damn well that they couldn't defeat someone who refused to give up. But my persistence was never about winning or proving anything to them. I stayed because I was fighting for something much deeper and more personal. I was doing it for me! It was about proving to myself that I was capable and good enough. Moreover, I was also doing it for every other woman who had faced similar struggles and felt the same sense of hopelessness and defeat. I wanted to be a beacon of strength and resilience, showing them that it was possible to persevere and thrive in the face of overwhelming odds.

It wasn't for nothing; I wouldn't allow it to be! Throughout my ordeal, I would catch glimpses of the bigger picture and intuitively knew my pain had to serve a purpose. For that to be realized, I had to make the conscious choice to pick myself up and confront everything head-on in order to truly heal. All the struggles and experiences I endured were not forms of punishment; they were essential preparation. Each challenge I faced, every moment of doubt, and every ounce of pain had forged me into a stronger, more resilient person.

When I viewed my experiences through a lens of gratitude and compassion toward myself, I couldn't help but acknowledge the undeniable truth staring me in the face. Despite the hardships, fear, and devastation I endured, I recognized that I wouldn't be where I am today without those experiences. Had I not gone through what I did, I wouldn't be able to make the impact I have been making today. My personal experiences have given me a depth of understanding and empathy that certifications and training alone could never provide. While my formal education and professional development have been valuable, nothing compares to the insights and capabilities I've gained from living through and overcoming such profound challenges.

I've been in the trenches, facing the darkest moments and nearly drowning in adversity. Yet I managed to pull myself out, clean myself off, and transform my pain into a powerful tool for change. This personal journey has become my driving force, my purpose. Because of what I've lived through, I can connect with others on a completely different level. I can offer guidance and support rooted in genuine experience, showing them that it's possible to overcome even the most daunting obstacles. My struggles have equipped me to lead others through their own challenges and demonstrate that resilience and recovery are within reach. Ultimately, my journey has not just been about surviving, but thriving and using my experiences to uplift others. I am committed to helping those who are still in the trenches, showing them that they, too, can emerge stronger and more empowered.

CHAPTER 39

More Than A Few Good Men

The villains didn't win. In my story, they never stood a chance. Though they played crucial roles, shaped the narrative and presented plenty of challenges, they ultimately served to highlight my strength and resilience. Without their presence, I wouldn't have ended up where I did. Their actions and opposition were the tests in which my character was forged, and they contributed greatly to the rich tapestry of my experiences. Yet where there was evil and darkness, there was always light.

I didn't paint everyone with the same brush. Yes, there were some extremely toxic and downright evil men in the department, but I never let their actions or behaviors color my perception of the others. There were more than a few exceptional men whose solid leadership I had the honor of working under, as well as alongside some truly incredible men I was proud to call my brothers. Outside of work, I considered them my friends. These were men who stood in their values, morals, and integrity and who treated everyone, including me, with respect. They led by example and never hesitated to lend a helping hand or get their hands dirty, regardless of rank. These men understood the assignment!

I valued and appreciated the good ones. Although I did express my gratitude to them, they may never have fully understood the depth of their impact on my career, and on me personally. I firmly believe that people need to feel appreciated, trusted, and respected. While I didn't always convey that in words, I discovered that the quickest way to these men's hearts was through their stomachs with treats. I was never shy about volunteering to sweeten them up and often brought in goodies or snacks. This small gesture was my way of showing them how much their support and camaraderie meant to me.

I had the pleasure of working on a couple of crews that were exceptionally fun and filled with lighthearted banter. I thrived in this atmosphere as it allowed me to be myself. I loved their quick wit and sharp comebacks! It was a place of fair play, where you had to be able to dish it out and take it in equal measure. I genuinely looked forward to going to work when I was part of these crews. The camaraderie and acceptance I experienced made every shift enjoyable and memorable. Some of my fondest and most cherished memories are from those times filled with laughter and shared experiences. Being included and accepted by my peers was all I had ever truly wanted, and on those crews, I found that sense of belonging.

I was hired by a man who had the courage to stand up for what he believed was right, even if it meant facing widespread animosity. He was a leader who didn't shy away from controversy or opposition; instead, he confronted it head-on. Despite the immense backlash, he made a bold decision to go against them and give me a chance. He was honest and upfront and told me that it wouldn't be easy, but he had complete faith in my abilities and was willing to navigate through the difficult journey with me. This man took a significant risk by bringing me on board. As expected, he endured criticism and resistance from some members. He proved to me that his concern for my well-being and safety was paramount. He earned my trust by being a man of his word and always following through on the promises he made to me. His door was always open when I needed it. Even though he was my boss, he always offered a space where our conversations could be candid and without judgement, and I could seek guidance and express my thoughts freely. He listened attentively and valued my input, which made me feel heard and understood, like an integral part of the team. I deeply respected him both as a man and as a leader. I will be forever grateful for the opportunity to have worked on his team and for the confidence he placed in me. His influence left a lasting impact on my professional journey and personal growth.

The first captain I had the honor of working under always treated me with respect and kindness. When he discovered my interest in becoming a firefighter, he did something unexpected; he befriended me. Unlike many others in the department, he encouraged me to follow my dream and welcomed me with open arms. He faced a gross amount of inappropriate teasing from some of his colleagues for that, but he truly didn't give a fuck about the opinions of others when it came to doing what he believed was right. He was a man of contradictions, extremely stubborn with a quick temper, yet remarkably patient with me. He humored me, answered all my questions and engaged in every possible conversation about firefighting. He was at his happiest when I sought his knowledge and relished the opportunity to share his expertise. The wealth of wisdom he imparted to me was invaluable and I deeply appreciated every lesson he taught. Many didn't know, but his heart was enormous; he cared deeply for the people in his life. He went above and beyond for me and my family and performed countless acts of kindness without ever being asked, never expecting anything in return. When I was home with a newborn and my husband was away working, he took it upon himself to look after us in the harsh winter months. He would show up like clockwork to handle the snow removal. His consistent and timely visits ensured that my driveway was always clear, and it gave me such peace of mind. Whether it was to allow me to get out in case of a medical emergency or simply to fetch supplies, he ensured I was able. His generosity and selflessness marked him as a truly good human. Starting my career under his leadership was truly an honor, and I am forever grateful for his guidance, support, and friendship. Rest in peace, Captain Hess.

The captain who let me drive the truck when I was only an auxiliary played a pivotal role in the early stages of my career. During the short time I had the privilege of working with him, he demonstrated immense patience and dedication, and took it upon himself to teach me the intricacies of the fire trucks and their operations. I had an obvious lack of mechanical inclination, but he had a remarkable talent for breaking down complex concepts into terms I could easily understand. He didn't just teach; he would test my knowledge and then celebrate my successes. That reflected him as a true leader and helped me feel proud of my achievements. He took the time to ensure I was included and was willing to give me a chance. He had a sharp wit, was funny as fuck, and was not afraid to get into a little trouble. He would often make light-hearted comments that had us all laughing. He would joke about how, back in the day, they had to sneak women into the firehall, but now they just provided them. I never took offence because I truly enjoyed his humor, and he was genuinely kindhearted. His ability to balance being a mentor and a leader made learning from him an enjoyable and enriching experience. His efforts left a lasting impact on me, and I am deeply thankful for the laughs we shared and the lessons I learned from one of the greats.

Throughout my career, I had the opportunity to work with various crews and was proud to serve alongside some truly remarkable firefighters. These men were not only exceptionally skilled and intelligent, but also profoundly honest and trustworthy. Our job often involved life-and-death situations that demanded unwavering teamwork and solid, trusting relationships. These men exemplified what it meant to be part of the brotherhood. Their abilities and dedication to their roles instilled a deep sense of confidence and security in me. I never had to question whether I could rely on them because their actions consistently demonstrated their commitment to our shared values and responsibilities. In the face of danger, I trusted these men with my life. Their professionalism and integrity made it easy to do so. They embodied the essence of what it means to be a firefighter and took their duties seriously and always prioritized the safety and well-being of the team. Their influence extended beyond their technical skills. They showed me that the true spirit of the brotherhood was more than just a professional network; it was also a circle of friends. I cared deeply not only for those brave men but also for their families. We were a professional community that looked out for one another, but also understood that our connections ran deeper than our duties. Our shared commitment to each other's well-being fostered a sense of unity and mutual support, creating a tight-knit family amongst some of us within the department. These men were not merely colleagues to me but individuals I held in high regard and with whom I shared a bond. Our connection extended beyond the fire station and encompassed genuine friendships that were built on trust, respect, and shared experiences. It was an honor to be part of such a remarkable group of individuals.

The one that changed everything for me was right at the tail end of my career. It was without a doubt the best working environment I had experienced the entire time I was there. The crew was led by exemplary leadership whom I deeply respected and valued. I was treated as an equal, included and accepted, and for the first time I felt like I truly belonged. I thrived in this setting! I was no longer nervous or scared and was able to perform my job to the best of my ability. Having a leader who nurtured my potential while trusting and believing in me changed everything. The atmosphere was filled with laughter, friendly wagers, and a sense of camaraderie that made me feel safe to be myself. This captain always led by example and constantly challenged me to step outside my comfort zone, which gave me the courage to trust myself. This shift in mindset revolutionized how I approached each day at work. He consistently demonstrated his belief in his team, often taking the time to mentor and encourage each member personally. Knowing that he unequivocally had my back—unlike the captain who told me I was on my own—he was a much-needed dose of security that allowed me to push my limits and excel. I was finally given the opportunity to prove my capabilities to myself before my career concluded, and I made sure I told him how profoundly grateful I was.

My father, though undoubtedly one of my biggest supporters, also played a role in the emotional turmoil I faced throughout my life. It took me a long time to acknowledge this truth and accept that I had always sought his approval. Some time ago I chose to distance myself and only allow access to my life on my terms. I could no longer tolerate the selfishness that often seeped into our relationship, so I learned the importance of firm boundaries. Our relationship has been a work in progress—a project of continual but minimal effort.

My father is a good man, and I love him deeply. His actions weren't rooted in malice, but in his own conditioning—a learned behavior that shaped a love that has often felt conditional and tied to achievement and obedience. Despite the challenges, I've gained valuable lessons through my experiences with my father—the most pivotal was making the decision to end the cycle of generational trauma that had flowed through our family. I chose to break the patterns that had shaped not just his life, but mine as well. This realization has driven me to do the hard work of healing my wounds and ensuring that I create corrective experiences for my own son. I'm committed to nurturing a healthy and loving environment for him, one that I wish had existed for me.

There will always be work to do—to right the wrongs I've carried forward from the messaging I received growing up. But ultimately, it stops with me.

I've chosen to break the chain.

In doing so I've ensured that the lessons passed down through my father's actions lead to growth and healing, not further pain. I am grateful for the strength that has come through both the love and the struggles of our relationship.

Three years before I retired from the fire department, I confronted my husband with brutal honesty and lay bare the reality of what had been happening between us in our marriage.

It was the most difficult conversation I had ever faced in a relationship. For a long time, things had been far from good. I had endured his behaviors and mistreatment just as I had with the men at the fire department. I found myself surrounded by men who took me for granted and abused their power in my presence. It was pervasive, so the fact that it was happening at home, too, seemed almost inevitable. But I had reached my breaking point. Home had to be the first place where I put my foot down and demanded better.

As I sat him down, my heart pounded, and my voice trembled with the weight of what I was about to say. This wasn't just about airing grievances; it was about reclaiming my self-respect and setting a new standard for how I deserved to be treated. I explained to him how his actions had eroded my trust and happiness, and how I could no longer accept the status quo. The patterns of mistreatment I had tolerated for so long had to end, and it had to start with him. I told him about the parallels between his behavior and that of my colleagues, making it clear that the change needed to begin at home.

I spoke and, thankfully, he listened. He accepted the truth and acknowledged his role in the deterioration of our relationship, vowing to make the necessary changes to be better. From that moment on, I witnessed a profound transformation in the man I thought I knew. He accepted full responsibility for his actions and behaviors and committed to a journey of self-improvement.

Day by day, he took deliberate and meaningful steps toward change. He sought therapy to understand the root of his actions, read books on personal growth, and actively participated in open and honest conversations with me about our future. He followed through on every promise he made, demonstrating his commitment not just through words, but through consistent and tangible actions.

What was even more remarkable was his willingness to give himself permission to evolve into the best version of himself. He shed old habits and embraced new, healthier ways of being. He became more attentive, compassionate, and considerate not just to me, but to our son and in all other aspects of his life.

Watching him grow was inspiring. It was a testament to the power of accountability and the capacity for change when one is truly committed. Our marriage, once teetering on the brink, began to flourish anew. He became a partner I could trust, respect, and love more deeply than ever before.

He had always stood by me, but never in the way he was showing up for me now. The qualities I had believed in and seen within him from the beginning were finally shining through. He had transformed into the loving, caring, and supportive partner I desperately needed.

This transformation did not happen overnight. It took a couple of years of relentless effort and corrective experiences for both of us. There were many moments of blood, sweat, and tears. It demanded deep levels of honesty and acceptance, hard work, and unwavering love. The journey was anything but easy, but it was undeniably worth it. His transformation was not just for the sake of our relationship but for himself as well. Ultimately, he grew into a more fulfilled and authentic version of who he was meant to be.

I am immensely proud of him and everything he has accomplished. He made the conscious choice to change, and because of that decision, he became a better father, a better husband, and ultimately a better man.

To the greatest man I'll ever know, my son.

From the moment you came into my life, you became my guiding light and my greatest motivation. Balancing the demanding roles of being a firefighter and a mother often seemed impossible and there were many times when I felt as though I was failing at both. There were days when the weight of my responsibilities seemed overwhelming, and I undoubtedly fell short on more occasions than I can count. Yet every time I stumbled, it was your sweet face that gave me the strength and reminded me of my purpose so I could get back up and keep going. It may have been hard to understand, but the sacrifices I made—the long hours, the missed moments, the physical and emotional toll—were all for you.

I know there were times when you needed me and I wasn't there because duty called. Those sacrifices were incredibly hard, and I often struggled with guilt. But every shift I took, every emergency I responded to was driven by my desire to make an impact in the world and ensure I could financially provide a stable home life at the same time. I also know there were many times when you needed me and I wasn't emotionally available. For many years the stress and demands of my job often left me exhausted and distant and for that I am truly sorry. My absence, both physically and emotionally, was never because I didn't care, but because I was stretched far too thin, trying to be everything for everyone else.

I deeply regret the moments when I reacted out of my own fears, weaknesses, and insecurities, and the times when I was mean, projecting my frustrations onto you because I lacked the strength to confront those who truly deserved it. I carried a lot of pain within me. Despite my best efforts, I couldn't always conceal it from you or shield you from its impact. Your perceptiveness and sensitivity have always astounded me; you've always had an incredible ability to sense when I needed compassion and unconditional love. In those moments, you have shown me an abundance of both, more than I could have ever hoped for or deserved. I want you to know that my actions were never a reflection of my feelings toward you but rather a manifestation of my own internal struggles. You have been a beacon of light in my darkest times and remained my greatest source of strength and inspiration.

Through all the challenges, my hope has always been to teach you some valuable lessons. I hope you've learned the importance of resilience, that no matter how many times life knocks you down, you have the strength to get back up. I hope you've seen the value of dedication and hard work, and how committing to something greater than yourself can bring immense fulfillment. I hope you understand the significance of compassion and service. Every day on the job, I tried to make a difference in someone's life, and I hope that spirit of helping others has inspired you. But above all, I hope for you to have courage. Courage to face challenges head-on, to stand up for what you believe in, and to never shy away from doing what's right, even when it's difficult. Courage to be yourself, to pursue your dreams, to speak your truth, and to embrace both the successes and failures that come your way.

You are my greatest achievement and my deepest pride. Watching you grow into the compassionate, brave, and intelligent young man you are today has been the most rewarding experience of my life. I see in you all the qualities of an amazing man—someone who is kind, strong, and unafraid to face the world head-on. As you continue to grow and find your path, know that it's okay to fail and to struggle. These moments do not define you; it's how you rise from them that truly matters. You have already shown incredible drive, strength and resilience, and I have no doubt you will continue to do so.

Thank you for choosing me to be your mother and for being my inspiration and my reason to strive to be better each day. I am endlessly proud of you, my special guy, and I love you with all my heart.

CHAPTER 40

It Worked—Until It Didn't

From the very start of my career, I was diligent about maintaining healthy coping mechanisms to manage the mental demands of my job. Understanding the potential psychological impacts that came with being a firefighter, I made a conscious effort to stay attuned to my mental health. I paid close attention to my reactions following every stressful or abnormal call, recognizing that each incident had the potential to affect me in different ways. By actively monitoring my emotional and mental state, I could be proactive in addressing any noted signs of distress with a variety of healthy coping strategies I employed.

I had always been extremely physically active, and the gym had always served as my sanctuary. It was a place where I could channel any mental or emotional burdens—whether a full head or a heavy heart—and work through them. The act of exercising allowed me to process and release stress, leaving me feeling lighter and more centered each time I walked out. In many ways, the gym was my therapy, a crucial outlet that kept my mental health in check and prevented me from spiraling. Fitness was not just about lifting weights or running miles; it was a holistic approach that encompassed nutrition as well. I was diligent about eating healthy and mindful of what I put into my body, treating it like a finely tuned machine. This attention to diet complemented my physical efforts and I took pride in maintaining a physique that reflected my commitment. While I admittedly had a bit of a sweet tooth and enjoyed social drinking, I believed in the principle of moderation and balance. These small indulgences were part of a broader, disciplined lifestyle that prioritized overall well-being without becoming restrictive.

Since a very young age, I have always loved to write. Whether it was poetry, short stories, or even letters to people—yes, old-school handwritten letters that I would mail—I found immense joy in the act of writing. To me, the connection in letter writing has become a lost art. Writing has always provided me with solace. While I only took up journaling later in life, it quickly became a healthy and safe space for me to process and release my experiences. There's something profoundly therapeutic about putting pen to paper. It felt like a dance, with rhythm and flow, allowing my deepest, darkest thoughts to pour out without hesitation. Journaling offered me a judgment-free zone where I could truly bear my soul. It was a place of total honesty, free from the fear of repercussions. Many times, after filling the pages with my innermost thoughts, I would shred or burn them to ensure they never fell into the wrong hands. Writing has been a constant companion throughout my life, providing an outlet for creativity and a means of emotional release. It's a practice that has allowed me to navigate the complexities of my thoughts and feelings with a deep level of honesty and self-reflection.

Journaling became a sanctuary where I could share my truth and confront the horrific details of my job. It served as a confidential outlet for the intense and often disturbing experiences I encountered on calls and allowed me to meticulously sort out the facts of what I had witnessed. This analytical approach—focusing strictly on the facts and avoiding the creation of any additional narratives—was something I excelled at. By dissecting the tiniest details and piecing together the fragments of each incident, I could process the calls methodically and ensure I did not carry their emotional weight with me. This practice was not just therapeutic; it was an essential tool that I relied on daily to maintain my mental clarity and emotional well-being. Journaling provided a structured way to handle the chaos and trauma of my work and enabled me to clear my mind and keep a balanced perspective. It was a disciplined routine that allowed me to unload my burdens and continue performing my duties with a clear head. Without a doubt, this practice played a crucial role in preserving my mental health and helping me navigate the disturbing nature of my profession.

I was no stranger to counseling and therapy. These resources played a pivotal role in helping me navigate various aspects of my life. I had the good fortune of having a trusted therapist even before I began my career, and I frequently turned to her for support after particularly tough calls. However, as I faced more intense and traumatic experiences, I realized that my therapist's expertise in trauma was limited. Understanding the importance of specialized support, I sought out a new therapist who had extensive experience in dealing with trauma. This transition was crucial, as it connected me with someone who could effectively guide and support me through the complexities of my profession. This new therapist provided the specific tools and insights I needed to manage the severe stress and emotional toll of my work. Her expertise allowed me to delve deeper into my experiences, ensuring I processed them in a healthy and constructive manner.

Of course, my most trusted source for talk therapy was my mother. She was my safest haven, a place where I could spill everything without fear of judgment. Knowing me better than anyone else, she could offer the best advice precisely when I needed it, or simply be a comforting presence when no words were necessary. My mother had an uncanny ability to talk me off the proverbial ledge and provided a calming influence during my most turbulent moments. Her wisdom and unconditional support were invaluable and served as my anchor when I felt overwhelmed by the demands and traumas of my job. She was my calm in the storm, offering a sense of stability and reassurance that no professional therapy could replicate. Our conversations often provided clarity and perspective, helping me to see beyond the immediate stress and find a path forward. Her innate understanding of my character and experiences allowed her to offer insights that were deeply personal and profoundly helpful. Whether I needed a sounding board for my thoughts, a compassionate ear, or a few wise words, my mother was always there, embodying the perfect balance of empathy and guidance. In many ways, she was my first and most enduring therapist, offering a level of emotional support that was unparalleled. Her role in my life was a cornerstone of my mental and emotional resilience and enabled me to navigate the challenges of my career and personal life with greater strength and confidence.

My healthy coping mechanisms were effective—until they weren't. Initially, I failed to recognize the situation for what it truly was; instead, I made excuses and rationalized almost everything. In hindsight, I see that I had suppressed emotions and experiences so deeply that even my rigorous workouts couldn't reach them. My body was constantly filled with tightness and tension, but I dismissed it as mere soreness from exercise. I didn't notice that my workouts were deteriorating—becoming less intense and shorter in duration. My drive and motivation were dwindling, and I had very little energy to give when I was at the gym. Additionally, I overlooked the fact that my diet had taken a nosedive, and every night consisted of chips, dip, and a bottle of wine as I watched mindless television. This phase extended for quite some time, during which my junk food and alcohol consumption spiraled out of control and lead to significant weight gain. I somehow managed to conceal these changes from others to some extent but photos didn't lie. When I finally looked back at them, I was horrified by what I saw. The evidence of my decline was unmistakable, starkly contrasting with the image of health and discipline I once maintained.

I continued journaling, but the focus of my entries had drastically shifted. Gone were the days when I chronicled the calls I responded to, the scenes I witnessed, and the tasks I performed at work. My journal had become a detailed record of the things said to me, said about me, and done to me. I meticulously documented the mistreatment, bullying, misogyny, and harassment I experienced for reasons I couldn't fully understand. There were numerous instances when I felt like I was losing my mind because colleagues would insist that certain incidents hadn't occurred. But each time I doubted myself, I would refer to my journal. There, in black and white, were the accounts of those very incidents. My journal had transformed into a tool for validating my sanity amid the gaslighting and chaos that some of my colleagues and bosses inflicted. It was a lifeline, confirming that my experiences were real and not figments of my imagination. Reading through hundreds of pages of these facts became a regular practice. It was a necessary exercise to navigate the chaos and often toxic work environment and remind myself that I wasn't going crazy. The act of journaling and revisiting these entries helped me maintain a grip on my sense of self and truth amidst the disorienting mind fuck that seemed all too common in my workplace.

I continued to see my therapist regularly and even she was horrified by the stories I shared with her—though I held back much of what I was experiencing. Her office provided a safe space where I could openly discuss the mistreatment I endured. She offered me tools and strategies to stand up for myself, emphasizing the importance of setting boundaries and recognizing abuse and manipulation. I always left feeling empowered, but it was short-lived. When it came down to it, I was always too afraid to implement any of her advice. The thought of standing up for myself felt daunting, and I lacked the courage to put her suggestions into practice. Each session, she assigned me homework designed to help me build resilience and assertiveness, but I never followed through. Instead, I used our sessions primarily as a space to vent my frustrations.

My healthy coping mechanisms and vigilant awareness for potential signs of post-traumatic stress disorder (PTSD) were effective in managing the stressors associated with my job. But when it came to the targeted bullying, discrimination, harassment, and misogyny, my coping techniques fell short. The personal nature of these attacks required a different set of tools and strategies—ones that I had not yet developed. I naively tried to apply the same coping strategies to both professional challenges and personal mistreatment, but this approach failed miserably. I attempted to lump all my experiences together, thinking that my established coping mechanisms would suffice. This miscalculation left me ill-equipped to handle the emotional and psychological toll of the personal mistreatment. Instead of resolving my issues, my efforts to use a one-size-fits-all approach only compounded my stress and suffering.

I never received an official PTSD diagnosis from a medical professional but the suffering I endured was immense and very real. The absence of a formal diagnosis stemmed from my narrow focus of the "on the job" perspective. I evaluated my symptoms solely in relation to work-related incidents, which meant I didn't meet the clinical criteria.

Certain details from some of the calls lingered or replayed in my mind, but typically only for a short period. Most often, these memories faded within a week. Occasionally, something I had seen, smelled, or heard would trigger a recollection and bring back snippets of a call, but these moments were fleeting. I never experienced full-fledged flashbacks. I was well-versed in the criteria for PTSD, and I knew that for a diagnosis, symptoms must persist for longer than thirty days. Since my symptoms didn't meet this duration, I dismissed the possibility of having PTSD.

I was so focused on one aspect of my life—the calls I responded to—that I developed tunnel vision and failed to consider anything outside of that scope. I was struggling and suffering, exhibiting a multitude of signs and symptoms, but I dismissed them because they weren't related to the calls. I hadn't even considered the personal attacks, threats, and bullying from my colleagues and bosses as potential sources of trauma. Their mistreatment had become so ingrained in my daily experience that I accepted it as normal. The normalization of abuse stemmed from a lifetime of similar experiences. It was my "normal" growing up, it was my "normal" in some of my relationships, and it had become my "normal" at work. In my mind, there was nothing traumatic about what I perceived as routine. I was conditioned to accept mistreatment as a given, and this skewed perspective prevented me from recognizing the true impact it had on my overall health. This blindness to the broader sources of my distress meant that I couldn't see the full extent of my suffering. My rigid definition of what constituted trauma kept me from understanding that the hostile and abusive behavior I had endured was just as damaging, if not more so, than the calls I attended.

I was disconnected and dysregulated in every conceivable way, trapped in a perpetual state of trauma response. I lived in a constant cycle of fight, flight, freeze, and fawn. If it seems impossible to experience all these responses simultaneously, I assure you it is not only possible but also incredibly debilitating. Intrusive thoughts and flashbacks of my experiences with the men haunted me relentlessly. I could vividly replay entire scenarios like a movie—the conversations, the menacing looks, the sound of evil laughter. These memories were etched into my mind and replayed with a cruel persistence. To cope, I overworked myself, staying perpetually busy and distracted. My hyper-independence stemmed from a deep mistrust of everyone around me. I couldn't relax or sit still because I was plagued by constant worry. My hypervigilance was exhausting. I was easily startled and always on guard. I spent much of my time metaphorically running away, desperately trying to hide the internal war I was fighting. Sleep was elusive, interrupted by frequent nightmares, and when I did manage to rest, it was never restorative. Concentration was a struggle, with dense, heavy brain fog clouding my thoughts. I often joked about having "baby brain," even though my son was far beyond the infant and toddler stages. It was my way of reasoning my loss of memory. My emotional state was volatile. I experienced extreme anger outbursts, intense mood swings, and my tolerance for anything was minimal at best. I lived in a state of heightened stress and fear, and my body and mind were constantly on high alert. The reason for this relentless anxiety was clear: my life had been threatened, and my sense of security was shattered. I was traumatized and living in survival mode.

Then I was introduced to the complex post-traumatic stress disorder (CPTSD) criteria and was able to meticulously check off each symptom. I thought back to the requirement of symptoms lasting longer than thirty days for PTSD. Just one month—that was all it took. Yet I had been living in that state for over a decade! Without a doubt I was injured, but I had excused and justified my suffering because it had become my normal. For years, I barely functioned, often barely managing to push through each day. I adopted a façade and would "fake it until I made it," but the toll it took on me was immense. Realizing that I had needlessly suffered for so long was heartbreaking. I had convinced myself that my experience was normal, not recognizing the trauma for what it truly was. My life had been an unending cycle of stress and anxiety, shaped by the personal attacks, threats, and bullying I endured. I coped by suppressing my emotions, staying hyper-busy, and overworking myself—all the while struggling with constant intrusive thoughts, flashbacks, and nightmares. My hyper-independence and inability to trust others were survival mechanisms in a world where I felt perpetually unsafe. I don't know how I managed to carry on, but somehow, I did. The realization that I had lived in survival mode for so long without recognizing or addressing the magnitude of my suffering was a brutal awakening.

One day, my mother and I were discussing PTSD and she candidly told me that she knew I had it. She was fully aware of everything I had endured and saw the impact those experiences had on me over the years. Being the closest person to me, she had a front-row seat to my struggles and the toll they took on my mental and emotional well-being. Would I have believed her if she had tried to intervene earlier? Absolutely not. I wasn't receptive at the time and would have resisted any attempts to address the issue. I believe she understood this instinctively. So instead of pushing the matter, she chose to stay close, keeping a watchful eye on me and always being there when I needed her. She recognized that coming to terms with my post traumatic struggles was something I had to do on my own. Deep down, she knew I needed to admit it to myself before I could accept help from others. Her approach was to provide unwavering support and unconditional love and be a constant presence in my life without pressuring me. She stood by me, ready to back me up in my fight, even though I never truly stepped into the ring.

I can only imagine how difficult it must have been for her to watch her child struggle and suffer, feeling powerless to fix things. Despite this, she did exactly what I needed her to do. For her patience, understanding, and support, I am forever grateful. She gave me the space to come to terms with my truths in my own time while ensuring I never felt alone. Her presence was a silent strength and a steady reassurance that no matter how tough the battle, she was right there with me.

My only regret is that I didn't recognize the signs earlier, sparing myself and those close to me from prolonged, unnecessary suffering. The realization that my family and friends had to endure the darker sides of my struggle—the volatile moods, the anxiety, the detachment—brings me immense pain. It wasn't fair to any of us. Reflecting on this, I see how deeply my untreated trauma affected those around me. They witnessed my emotional turmoil and bore the brunt of my outbursts and unpredictable behavior. Their patience and love were stretched thin, yet they stood by me, most often without fully understanding what I was going through. The burden I unknowingly placed on them fills me with regret.

Trauma is the disconnection from self—a fracture in the mind, body and spirit that left me feeling isolated, fragmented, and lost within my own life. It severed the bond between who I was and who I believed I could be, leaving me stranded in a state of survival. Healing on the other hand, is the slow, delicate process of reconnection—of reclaiming parts of myself that were hidden away in the shadows of pain. It's the journey back to wholeness—a rediscovery of inner strength and self-compassion. I consider myself fortunate to have experienced post-traumatic growth, not because the trauma was any less painful, but because in the aftermath, I found new depths within myself. Through the struggle I was able to reconnect with a deeper sense of purpose, an expanded capacity for love, and a renewed perspective on life. The trauma may have disconnected me from my true self, but in healing, I was able to rebuild, becoming not just who I was before, but someone more resilient, wiser, and more grounded in my own truth.

CHAPTER 41

Mountains Can Be Moved

I truly believe there is a lesson embedded in every experience we encounter. At times, these lessons can be difficult to recognize or comprehend—especially when we're in the thick of challenges. But regardless of how elusive they may seem, they are always there, waiting to be acknowledged. It took me a long time to realize that the same situations kept resurfacing in my life, not because of coincidence, but because I wasn't grasping the lesson being offered. I found myself stuck in a cycle—swearing I had already dealt with the repetitive issue—but there it was again. It wasn't until I got really fucking honest and took a step back to reevaluate what I was missing, and what was really happening, that I began to see clearly. Once I embraced this shift, I was able to heal and evolve.

Through my painful journey I have learned to fully appreciate the wisdom hidden in each experience and move forward with a deeper understanding of myself and the world around me.

1. *Self-awareness and early intervention are crucial for good mental health*: I've learned the crucial importance of being attuned to my mental health. Recognizing the early signs of distress—such as persistent sadness, anxiety, or feeling overwhelmed—has been vital. Seeking help sooner rather than later can prevent years of unnecessary suffering. Through my experiences, I've realized that brain health is just as important as physical health, and early intervention can make a significant difference.

Acknowledging when I need help and reaching out for it has been a powerful step toward healing and maintaining my well-being.

2. *The impacts of trauma are far-reaching*: Trauma doesn't just affect the individual; its ripples extend to everyone around them. This awareness has deepened my empathy and understanding toward others' struggles. I've witnessed how trauma can shape behaviors, relationships, and perspectives. It has taught me to approach people with greater compassion, recognizing that everyone carries unseen burdens. Understanding the wide-reaching impact of trauma has made me more patient and considerate, knowing that a kind word or a listening ear can make a profound difference in someone's life.
3. *Understand the significance of support systems*: My support system, though small, has been incredibly mighty. This group provided me with a foundation of unwavering support, teaching me the power of patience, love, and resilience. Their presence highlighted the importance of having a strong support network to pick me up when I had fallen. Through their support, I've learned that no one should have to face challenges alone. The strength and stability they offered helped me navigate through difficult times and reinforced the value of who I surround myself with. This experience has underscored the critical role of community and connection in personal growth and recovery.
4. *Speak your truth*: Through my experiences, I've realized the immense value of honesty. It's not only about being truthful to others; it's also about being true to myself. Speaking my truth—even when my voice shakes—means

acknowledging my feelings, desires, and needs without fear. It's about shedding the masks I wore to fit in or to be accepted. In speaking my truth, I've found a sense of liberation and authenticity that allows me to live more genuinely.

5. *Practice self-compassion*: I've learned the importance of being gentle with myself, especially when facing challenges or reflecting on past mistakes. Self-compassion means offering myself the same kindness and understanding that I would offer a small child. It's about recognizing that everyone makes mistakes and it's okay to be imperfect. Through self-compassion, I've learned to forgive myself and to nurture my well-being. This practice has allowed me to grow and heal in ways I never thought possible.
6. *Establish boundaries*: Setting healthy boundaries has been an often uncomfortable but crucial lesson. It's about understanding that my time, energy, and emotions are valuable. Establishing boundaries means saying no when necessary and not overextending myself to please others. It's about acknowledging what brings me joy and protecting my peace at all costs. Boundaries are for protection, not punishment. I've realized that they are not about keeping people out, but about ensuring that the relationships I have are respectful and mutually beneficial. By doing so, I've created a healthier and more balanced life.
7. *Stand in your power*: This lesson is about recognizing and embracing my own strength and capabilities. I've learned to trust in my abilities and to stand firm in my decisions and beliefs. Standing in my power means not allowing others to diminish my worth or dictate my path. It's about

being confident in who I am and what I can achieve. This empowerment has given me the courage to pursue my goals and dreams unapologetically.

8. *Don't keep secrets to keep others comfortable*: By not keeping secrets for the sake of others, I learned the profound value of honesty and authenticity. This lesson was very challenging, but it taught me that the discomfort of truth is an act of vulnerability that empowered me to take back control of my narrative. Releasing the burden allowed me to stop owning other people's actions and sacrificing my own well-being. It rebuilt my self-confidence, self-trust, and freed the shame and guilt that consumed me. Doing this created space for deeper understanding, genuine relationships, and personal growth.
9. *The disapproval of others is theirs, not yours*: This insight has been liberating. I've come to understand that criticism and disapproval from others often stem from their own unresolved issues and insecurities. Their negative opinions do not define my value or my choices. By internalizing this lesson, I've learned not to take such disapproval personally. Instead, I focus on my journey and trust in my decisions, knowing that I am not responsible for others' actions or insecurities. This realization has freed me from the burden of seeking external validation and has strengthened my self-confidence.
10. *Sacrificing your voice for peace isn't true peace*: Sacrificing my voice to maintain peace was not an honorable exchange because I never reaped true peace. I was left with uncomfortable silences and resentment as I watched others feel better because of my martyrdom. If I must

silence my thoughts, feelings, or beliefs to avoid conflict, the resulting peace is superficial and unsustainable. True peace involves open communication, mutual respect, and the freedom to express oneself. By honoring my voice, I foster genuine and lasting harmony in my relationships.

11. *Fear is a liar*: Fear is a liar, and it only keeps me small. Fear often whispers falsehoods that limit my potential and hold me back from pursuing my dreams. By recognizing fear for what it is—a barrier rather than a truth—I've been able to push past it and achieve things I once thought impossible. Embracing courage over fear has been crucial in my journey towards self-empowerment and personal growth.
12. *You're on your own*: No one was coming to save me. The strength I needed to heal, grow, and overcome was within me all along. I realized I couldn't find healing in the same place, and with the same people, that broke me. The pain of staying the same was far greater than the pain of change. I was just one decision away from transforming my life. So I chose to own my journey and ignite the fire within, stepping fully into my power.

I am grateful for the lessons learned. As hard as they were, they revealed that I possess an immense reservoir of courage and bravery, and my resilience is unparalleled. My psychological injuries were not a life sentence. I believed in my ability to overcome them and dedicated myself to the grueling work of healing. I was determined to break free from its grip. Throughout this journey, I discovered that I am unique in my capacity to stand in the flames of hardship, but I also have the power to step out when I choose to.

The darkest part of my story gave birth to the strongest part of my soul. I have grown into a more aware, compassionate, and resilient human being. Moving forward, I am committed to applying these lessons to live a healthier, more mindful life and to support others who might be on a similar journey. I am uniquely qualified to help the person I used to be, and without a doubt, I was given this mountain to show others that it can be moved.

"I survived because the fire inside me burned brighter than the fire around me."

—Joshua Graham

Acknowledgements

This book wouldn't have been possible without the support and belief from so many people. I knew I needed to write this book not only for me, but for all those who have ever kept secrets to keep others comfortable and sacrificed their wellbeing in the process. Thank you to everyone who believed in me—especially when I doubted myself—and encouraged me to share my story.

My incredible mother Debbie, who has been through it all with me. Thank you for your unwavering love, support and guidance throughout my life. You have always been my constant source of inspiration and comfort, and for that I am endlessly grateful. Your sacrifices and dedication have never gone unnoticed.

My amazing husband Wade, thank you for doing this life with me and choosing to face every challenge and every triumph together. We've been through a lot and you're always my constant. I appreciate you and I love you. Today. Tomorrow. Forever.

My brother Tanner, who at the time of publishing this book is celebrating 11 months of sobriety. Thank you for fighting for yourself and those you love. To say I'm proud of you is an understatement, and I am truly grateful for every hug I receive from you.

My business bestie Katie, who started out as my therapist and became one of my very best friends. You gave me a safe space to be myself, encouraged me to use my voice, and literally changed my life. You inspire me and push me to be the best version of myself. I am truly grateful for your friendship. I love you dude!

My bitches Nicki, Laurena, and Amanda, I love you all dearly. Thank you for coming into my life when I needed you the most and showing me what real ride-or-die friendship looks like. The laughter, the endless support, and the unfiltered group text make my life complete. Cheers to mimosas and more beach adventures bitchachos!

My editor Jenna, thank you for your guidance in bringing my words to life. Your sharp insights and attention to detail have elevated my work in ways I could never have achieved on my own. You pushed me to expand, and I am truly grateful for the impact you've had on this project.

My photographer Kimberly, thank you for capturing moments with such creativity, and always bringing my vision to life. I'm incredibly grateful for the magic you brought to the book cover, and my bio photo.

My family, friends, and clients who have followed me, supported me, and loved me through it all. Thank you for trusting me and navigating this journey with me. I see you, I support you, thank you, I love you.

About The Author

Lynnette Fritshaw is a retired career firefighter who dedicated eighteen years to the fire service, where she bravely faced the challenges of emergency response and the emotional toll that came with it. Now an entrepreneur, she is passionate about supporting others as they navigate crises and heal from trauma. Drawing from her unique experiences, she understands the struggles of those she seeks to assist, particularly the person she used to be.

Her memoir, You're On Your Own, reflects her journey of resilience and transformation, aiming to inspire others to confront their own challenges. With a deep commitment to self-empowerment, she encourages individuals to find their voice and share their stories, believing that vulnerability can lead to healing and connection.

Beyond her professional endeavors, Lynnette is a loving mother and wife, cherishing moments spent with her family. She resides in Alberta, Canada, with her husband and son. Through her work, she aspires to create a safe space for others to explore their narratives and embrace their journeys of recovery.

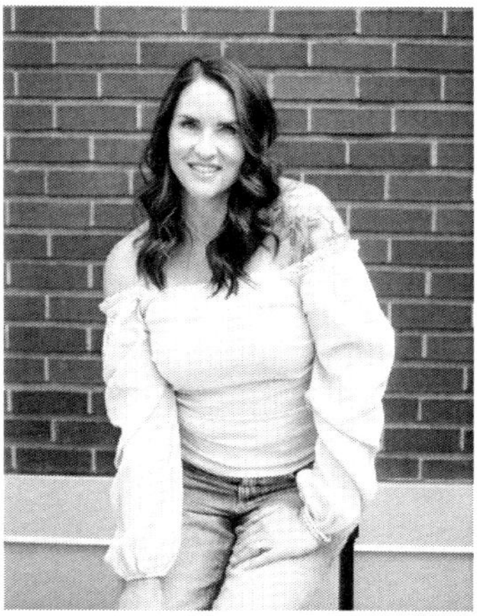

Connect with Lynnette:
www.firewithincrisisservices.com
Instagram @firewithincrisisservices

Made in United States
Cleveland, OH
15 February 2025

14370746R10201